'This book gives an important, valuable platform to many diverse trans voices. We must listen and learn from their experiences and concerns, and act in solidarity with their human rights struggle.'
— *Peter Tatchell, Director, Peter Tatchel Foundation*

'We congratulate Declan Henry on developing this perceptive account of trans experiences, richly illustrated with a wide array of authentic personal narratives. It is a timely reminder of the diversity of trans individuals and the many barriers to equal treatment they still face. We commend the book to everyone who is in a position to improve their lives.'
— *Bernard Reed, OBE, Trustee, Gender and Identity Research and Education Society (GIRES)*

'Declan Henry starts the book with a refreshingly honest confession that at one point he knew very little about the T in LGBT. With complete earnestness he sets out to give an overview of the transgender community in simple and very readable sections. He has packed this small book full of information, snippets of enlightening interviews and his thoughts about transgender equality and equality in its widest sense. A must-read for anyone wishing to be an ally who realises that only with knowledge and understanding can you change hearts and minds.'
— *Juno Roche, writer, campaigner and patron of cliniQ*

'Declan Henry's *Trans Voices* captures the diversity of the breadth of the transgender experience through personal stories that make the topic accessible and understandable for any reader and give the book heart that many other books on the subject lack.'
— *Charlie Craggs, Founder of Nail Transphobia*

TRANS VOICES

of related interest

Transitioning Together
One Couple's Journey of Gender and Identity Discovery
Wenn B. Lawson and Beatrice M. Lawson
ISBN 978 1 78592 103 2
eISBN 978 1 78450 365 9

Can I tell you about Gender Diversity?
A guide for friends, family and professionals
CJ Atkinson
ISBN 978 1 78592 105 6
eISBN 978 1 78450 367 3

TRANS VOICES
Becoming Who You Are

Declan Henry

Foreword by Professor Stephen Whittle, OBE
Afterword by Jane Fae

Jessica Kingsley *Publishers*
London and Philadelphia

First published in 2017
by Jessica Kingsley Publishers
73 Collier Street
London N1 9BE, UK
and
400 Market Street, Suite 400
Philadelphia, PA 19106, USA

www.jkp.com

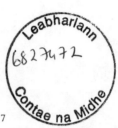

Copyright © Declan Henry 2017
Foreword copyright © Stephen Whittle 2017
Afterword copyright © Jane Fae 2017

Front cover image source: Gary Reddin.

Library of Congress Cataloging in Publication Data
A CIP catalog record for this book is available from the Library of Congress

British Library Cataloguing in Publication Data
A CIP catalogue record for this book is available from the British Library

ISBN 978 1 78592 240 4
eISBN 978 1 78450 520 2

Printed and bound in Great Britain

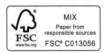

MIX
Paper from
responsible sources
FSC® C013056

This book is dedicated to my friend James

Contents

Interviewees

I interviewed several dozen trans people for this book. Many wished to be anonymous so their names and some other details have been changed.

Foreword

Professor Stephen Whittle, OBE
Press for Change, UK

Before starting this incredibly useful and often astonishing book by Declan Henry, I suggest you do the following (very small) exercise. Even if you have read Radclyffe Hall's lesbian novel *The Well of Loneliness*, but know little of the history surrounding it, just look it up on Wikipedia. Acquaint yourself with some of the furore that surrounded this rather worthy and somewhat dull book and the massively publicised 1928 obscenity trial which led to a ban on its publication or sale in Britain, for more than 20 years.

I was 15 when I managed to get hold of a copy of Hall's novel. I hoped it might carry some of the intensely erotic sexual desire described in D. H. Lawrence's *Lady Chatterley's Lover*. Lawrence's book had been the subject of an obscenity trial in 1960, but found by a jury to be unlikely to deprave the reader, despite its descriptions of sexual intercourse and many expletives such as f**k and c**t. Like so many teenagers, I had managed to read the well-thumbed copy of Lawrence's soap opera of Edwardian desire that had been passed around at school.

Disappointingly, there were no hot fumblings in the potting shed in *The Well of Loneliness*. Nowhere in Hall's story of her protagonist, Stephen Gordon, and his (her) quest for a lover and lifelong relationship, can we find anything that might be described as stimulating or suggestive. If you have read it, you will know the novel contains nothing which might raise your pulse rate, never mind set your loins aflame. The nearest inkling of any sexual activity between Stephen Gordon and Marym, the woman he loves, is in the one phrase:

...and that night, they were not divided.

That insinuates that they could have been up all night having a good gossip or a midnight feast, whilst playing canasta, which was the sort of thing my girlfriends and I did at Girl Guide camp.

I had hoped that Hall's thinly disguised semi-autobiographical account of hir love for a woman – note my careful use of the word 'hir' instead of her – would reflect something of my teenage angst. Stephen Gordon was a wo/man who loved and desired a woman. Being madly in love myself with a girl at one of Manchester's best all-girls schools, I hoped the novel would explain how and what I was meant to do with that love. I already knew it was a forbidden love; in 1970, for me, it was still a love without a name.

Comprehending Hall's novel was painful – it is very worthy, and written in a romanticised pastiche of Shakespeare's 16th century English – and very distressing. In a moment of clarity I realised I wasn't going to grow up to be a lesbian. Stephen Gordon's feelings were unmistakably descriptions of my own. This was a fictional account of my own sense of self-hood, and yet, despite the author's insistence at the obscenity trial that this was a book about lesbian love, it was – to me, at least – not an account of a woman in love.

To read *The Well of Loneliness* was to study the despair of a man who everyone else could only see as a woman. It was another breach in the dyke (pardon the pun). I came to realise that I had no choice but to try and find a way of getting the impossible, a sex change – or not to live at all.

At the obscenity trial, the judge decided that any literary merit of Hall's novel was irrelevant and what mattered was that: *No reasonable person could say that a plea for the recognition and toleration of inverts was not obscene.*

By 'inverts' the judge was clearly referring to us all: lesbian women, gay men and trans people; we were all lumped together because in 1928, the law, medicine and society had no doubt we were all the same.

Until the early 1970s, gay men, lesbian women and trans people found themselves locked in a set of assumption traps. The dominant assumption of heteronormativity as regards sexual orientation was that anyone born female who wished to dress in a masculine way, would only wish to do so in order to seduce another person born female, and anyone born male who wished to dress in a feminine way, would only wish to do so to be seduced by another person born male. As the judge said of Stephen Gordon, effectively Hall herself, in the *Wells* obscenity trial, L, G, B or T, we were all equally as disturbed and perverted, and, as 'inverts', not worthy of any form of defence.

Ever since the early medieval period, the law had not distinguished between people who loved members of their own sex group, and those who wanted to change sex groups and love someone of the (now) opposite sex. Until really quite recently, the criminalisation and persecution of gay men and lesbian women meant that those who could hide their sexuality would do so. But, for those who were trans, it was a much more difficult task. It was more than hiding your sexuality, it actually meant hiding your core self, the very person you are.

Until the mid-1930s, separation and analysis of the chemistry of sex hormones in the lab and the later scientific capabilities to replicate and manufacture them, to change sex was not only unattainable, but madness. In psychiatry, it was the same type of madness that makes people think they are Napoleon or Jesus, and therefore, some believe they are a man (or woman) in opposition to their birth and developed body. The same logic that made trans people the same sort of 'invert' as those who were gay or lesbian, would therefore label many gay men and lesbian women as being as mad as those misguided souls who wanted to change their sex.

I explain this partly because it shares a little about myself, but also because it describes just one of the many crossroads along the paths which lesbian, gay and trans people have travelled. Look closely and you will see that the paths have always been just that little bit separate and different yet, throughout our communities' histories, they have always been very much connected. Like tracing a Celtic knot, when studying L, G, B or T history, one can never be certain of which track one is following. You may cross over your own pathway, or that of another, or the paths may run alongside each other for a while, then criss-cross under the other's path, before apparently rejoining as you turn a corner. Along these pathways we have often held hands whilst travelling together in joint battles for equality, for liberty, for the right to be, for the right to love and for the right to be loved. These are the roads along which our community histories have been written, and the crossroads along the way have been the points at which we have been engaged together in our battles with the law.

People who are lesbian, gay, bi or trans have a great deal in common, not least our joint history of persecution, and yet many gay men and lesbian women still do not understand what it means to be trans. As trans people, whoever we love, or sleep with, our complex bodies complicate our sexualities. As a trans man, if I love a man there will be those who ask why I want to change my gender, and they clearly don't get it when I answer, 'What's my gender identity got to do with the gender of the person I love?'

Likewise, as a trans man, if I love a woman, then the same people would say that I must be a butch lesbian, who cannot live with the shame of my perverse sexual orientation. And again they don't get it when I say, 'What has the gender identity of the person I love got to do with my gender?' Either way, my sexuality or sexual orientation is never legitimate, so we do understand what it is like to be lesbian or gay, because, even with gender reassignment treatments and surgeries, our bodies will never lose the traces of our past, and our ways of being will never lose the traces of our upbringing and socialisation.

Now that many of the legal battles have been won, what many trans people would really like is a transformation in the dynamics of our relationship with the gay and lesbian communities – or as a trans woman once put it to me:

I would like gay and lesbian people to consider me desirable both in theory and in practice. I am not some jolly little mascot for the queer community, a person who will come and lip-sync to Judy Garland for their entertainment. When I go to a gay bar, I would like to have the same potential of finding love that all the other lesbian women in the room have.

And as a trans man, I agree.

Put another way, when I sit in an Equalities committee meeting, why do people assume the only things I know about, and should therefore restrict my remarks to, are trans issues? There is so much more to me than that – I can now discuss being older and disabled. I am of an indeterminate sexual or gender orientation (I am attracted by smiles – gender and genitals are irrelevant). Moreover, having been raised as a girl, I know what it is like not to naturally have the skills needed to dominate meetings in the way my male colleagues can, and I also know what it is like not to be believed, or taken seriously, after being a victim of sexual assault.

Being a trans activist, of course, I am able to contribute to the discussions of trans people's issues, but I am not some sort of trans person representative. When another trans person is nominated to the committee, I have heard it said that they are not needed as they already have me. But I am just one of many types of trans people; I lead just one sort of trans person's life.

Whether in my employment, my neighbourhood, the parent governor committee, the Pride committee or at a gay bar, I do want to be known as a trans person. But, I also want to be seen as a whole person. The same comes to making friends, forming relationships or just becoming someone's lover for one glorious night of passion. I want to have the same possible future, and be included in the battles and victories of life that everyone else in the room has.

So, if you find yourself fancying a trans person, don't run a mile. Do as you would with anyone else you fancy; date, laugh and become friends. Only if you decide to become lovers will you need to discuss body geographies. Without that chat, though, I am certain that if your desire makes you jump into bed with a trans person, those minor difficulties will be resolved in the heat of the moment.

Which brings me back to this book that Declan Henry has written for lesbian and gay communities. Declan has done a great job of writing a pithy, easily understood guide to the roadways within the Celtic knot along which L, G, B and T people now travel. The guide is written with a mature understanding of their hopes and fears, the actualities of trans people's lives, their bodies and the complex processes involved in becoming visible as their real, true selves. Effectively and efficiently, Declan has outlined and explained the project that trans people undertake simply in order to be. He explains the importance of the project to trans people, and how, for each of us, the project is slightly different.

Declan allows the voices of the many trans people he has interviewed to tell the blood and guts of the tale. It is highly readable, and compact enough in its clarity that it won't take up the rest of your life. It not only highlights the variety of trans people's lives and their battles with the world, but also the commonalities we have with gay and lesbian people in both our personal struggles and public campaigns. In the 19th century, we were all bundled together under the same mental health category of 'inverts'. In 2017 as L, G, B and T people, it becomes obvious that we need to undertake our political project together. Readers will begin to understand why trans people take on the long, hard project of such major personal change. Importantly, though, readers will see that trans people do so, in effect, for the same reasons that all people who want to develop and mature into a full life undertake their own small projects. Perhaps, the greatest thing every human being can learn in life is to give and receive love.

Acknowledgements

Sincere thanks to all of the wonderful interviewees featured in the book who provided me with great insight into both their own individual lives and that of trans issues.

I would also like to thank the many professionals who advised me, including James Morton from Scottish Transgender Alliance, Broden Giambrone from Transgender Equality Network Ireland (TENI), Professor Stephen Whittle, OBE from Press for Change and Bernard Reed from the Gender Identity Research and Education Society (GIRES). I would also like to give a special mention to Janett Scott from the Beaumont Society for her help, wit and charm.

Special appreciation to Gary Reddin (designer and illustrator) in Sligo for designing the striking jacket cover.

Lastly, many thanks to everyone at Jessica Kingsley Publishers, especially senior commissioning editor Andrew James, for his valued expertise and belief in the book.

INTRODUCTION

As a gay man, I decided to write this book because I was ashamed of how little I knew about trans people. Being part of the lesbian, gay, bisexual and transgender (LGBT) community, I regret that amongst the gay community there is still a general lack of knowledge about trans people and the issues they face on a day-to-day basis. In most Western countries, tolerance of gays and lesbians is greater than for trans people, who are still vilified and far more likely to be ostracised at work, beaten-up or in some countries even murdered. It is therefore reasonable to ask if trans people are the last group in society that can be ridiculed and judged without any apparent consequence.

How can society change its attitudes towards trans people? True equality isn't just about tolerance, because to imply that people simply ought to be tolerant towards trans people would mean that there is something wrong with them that needs control. What is needed is a broadminded and empathetic attitude, but this can't be achieved without understanding trans identities and dispelling the myths and fears about it; this was another reason for me writing about the subject.

In the chapters that follow, I will take the reader on a journey that shows the rich landscape of trans people, what it's truly like to be trans in today's world, and how the walls of suppression and secrecy around trans identities are steadily being torn down. It is my hope that, after you have finished reading this book, you will have a greater understanding of trans people and that, irrespective of whether or not you are part of the LGBT community, you are willing to be their ally and embrace their equality on the same level as you value your own. Equality for trans people can only be achieved when ignorance is challenged and stripped away.

In writing this book, my background as a qualified social worker helped me to find why there were women and men who felt uncomfortable in their gender and sought to change it. I interviewed dozens of trans people and found the accounts of their lives to be candid and often moving. Interviewing trans people for this book was a humbling experience and I learned so much about their lives. Although the people I interviewed were from ordinary backgrounds, they were extraordinarily brave people in the decisions they made to become the people they are today.

My brain tells me I am a man and that is how I live my life. How different it would be if it told me I was a woman and I was stuck in my male body. Who am I to say that I would put up with this predicament and not seek to change my gender to find the happiness and contentment that would otherwise have eluded me? Through my interviews I sought to gain a better understanding of trans people, including those who didn't consider themselves male or female, as in the case of non-binary people. I also wanted to explore and demystify the rationale behind cross-dressing.

There are as many differences as there are similarities between trans and gay people. Misconceptions and discrimination affect both, and they share similar nuances. They are closely acquainted in terms of homophobia and transphobia. Although homophobia is still prevalent in certain sections of Western culture, and whilst homosexuality is still illegal in over 75 countries, there is no denying that progress in terms of inclusion and acceptance is more commonplace than not, culminating in same-sex marriage legislation in many countries. Up until it was declassified in 1992, homosexuality was deemed a mental disorder under *psychiatric illnesses*. But trans people are still under the mental illness umbrella of psychiatry and have their own diagnostic criteria. Having a mental health label leads to society viewing trans people as being unwell, different or strange. For many years now, there has been visibility in the media about sexuality being on a continuum where no person is 100 per cent gay, or, indeed, 100 per cent heterosexual, and maybe everyone will find themselves somewhere on this continuum. This has prompted a lot of people to examine the way they view themselves, which, in turn, has encouraged acceptance of lesbian, gay and bisexual people.

It is only in very recent times that any similar visibility has started to emerge in regard to viewing gender as a continuum rather than a binary of just male or female, although it's commonly acknowledged that everybody has feminine and masculine characteristics irrespective of their gender. The chapters that follow outline the complexities of being transgender but ultimately they will show the simplicity of the situation – that a person is their self-identified gender even if this differs from the gender they were assigned at birth.

Nearly all the adults I interviewed noted that they had had issues with their gender identity in childhood. Many recalled how, as boys, they dressed as girls – and vice versa – and how, as children, they played with toys designed for the opposite sex. Some of them only felt comfortable playing with children of the opposite physical sex. These were childhoods filled with silence: how they felt about themselves was never discussed and only rarely were any of them able to confide in a family member or friend. So great was their distress about their bodies, their pubescent years were often marked by self-harming incidents and suicide ideation.

These days, however, gender identity problems in children are becoming more recognised than in previous generations, with many children having the confidence to speak out and say they do not self-identify with the gender they were assigned at birth. Children who do so may be prescribed hormone blockers in the early stage of puberty, but giving puberty blockers to children is controversial. Some argue that it is wrong to give powerful drugs to young people to suppress their puberty, whilst others, particularly observers of trans people who received puberty blockers in adolescence, have identified improved social integration and reduced mental health distress as positive outcomes of this treatment. Hormone blockers stop the body developing into an adult shape and delay the onset of puberty until the young person reaches 16 years of age, when she or he is deemed old enough to make an informed decision about whether to undergo masculinising or feminising hormonal treatment, although surgery is not offered before the age of 18.

This book is about adult trans people and covers many of the key areas and issues that affect the daily lives of trans people. Their views and opinions are paramount to the text. I think you will find their voices, outlining their thoughts and feelings, to be captivating and enriching.

I am aware that much curiosity surrounds trans people, and I too have bought into this. I know if I'm sitting next to a trans person in a restaurant or on a train it's enticing to look at their clothes, footwear and make-up, particularly if it's a trans woman. I have even found myself rooting for the person when they are spoken to by a waiter or a ticket collector – and when they get up and walk. I have wanted them to be convincing in their new gender because I know it's a harsh world and that people have a propensity for saying horrible things, shattering confidence and attacking self-worth in the process. But society doesn't have to be like this. I firmly believe that awareness and knowledge break down ignorance and bigotry and can create a world where everybody can get on with their business without interference or prejudice, thus allowing people to become whoever they want to be. Therefore, it is the voices in this book that will reach out to you when descriptions of their experiences are conveyed because they are coming from lived lives rather than from me as a mere spectator. Ultimately, I hope these voices will draw you closer to what it is like to be a trans person in today's world.

The transgender community comes with its own unique terminology. Although there is a full glossary at the back of the book which gives an overview of the main nomenclature, certain words and terms need clarification at this point if you are new to the subject. The word 'trans' is a shortened word for transgender, an umbrella term that comprises the identities and behaviours of a wide range of people who do not self-identify with the stereotypical man or woman binary categorisation of individuals into which they were assigned at birth. This includes those who don't identify as men or women but describe themselves as non-binary, as well as those who cross-dress. The term 'assigned at birth', which is used frequently throughout the book, is used by trans men, trans women and non-binary people to describe the inadvertent mistake they consider was made about their gender identity when they were born. The word 'cisgender' basically means somebody who is not a trans person.

CHAPTER ONE

BEING TRANS

Inside the trans world

The trans community is made up of a broad spectrum of gender nonconforming people. In describing this diverse community I will use the term 'gender identity' (who you know yourself to be), which may be as a man or woman or a mixture of both or neither. I recognise that individuals should be free to self-identify in any way they choose. However, for convenience, I have grouped the people whose voices I convey in this book as trans women, trans men, non-binary people and cross-dressing people. A trans woman is someone who was assigned male at birth but self-identifies as female and therefore transitions from male to female (MTF). Once transitioned, she may refer to herself as a woman with a trans history. A trans male is one who transitions in the other direction, from female to male (FTM). Once transitioned he may refer to himself as a man with a trans history. After transition, some men and women do not wish to disclose or ever refer to the fact that they have a trans history and this is sometimes referred to as 'being stealth'.

Laura, trans woman. 'It is like you've been wearing a really itchy suit your entire life and didn't know, until now, you could take it off. In the trans community we call normally gendered people cisgendered. Quite frankly, most of us would prefer to be that way given the choice. If we have the choice and luck to transition, then we too become cisgendered since our brain sex and physical sex are the same. What every trans person can say is that they just "know" their gender is wrong for their biological sex and that this has no bearing on sexual preference.'

It is important not to forget that being a trans person is entirely about gender and is independent of sexual orientation. Trans people can be lesbian, gay, bisexual or heterosexual, just like everybody else. These days, being trans is an issue that is steadily becoming more visible, more talked about and ultimately more acceptable, after centuries of suppression and denial.

Shirley, trans woman. 'As a teen in the '60s I thought I was homosexual. That was the definition given to us, and when I was old enough to search medical and psych books, I discovered I was a transvestite. Of course, that definition didn't fit either. I also discovered that treatment was with heavy psychotropic drugs, then electro shock therapy and finally lobotomy.'

Every year more and more trans people who previously felt too isolated and alone to admit the truth about who they are become more confident to declare their true identities. There is now more social exposure from social media, and the trans community is continuously gaining allies from this. The law now provides them with a large measure of protection. It is a big breakthrough for many, which has resulted in freedom from having to live a life that made them feel separated and different to other people.

Numbers

Whilst it is difficult to ascertain a true approximation of how many trans people there are in society, it is reasonable to assume that as the stigma crumbles a truer statistical picture will emerge. At the moment it is thought that trans people make up less than one per cent of the population, meaning that ten people out of every 1000 feel that the sex they were assigned at birth and the gender they identify with do not correspond.

New phenomenon?

There have been accounts of trans people since the beginning of recorded history. There are biblical quotes in Deuteronomy: *No one whose testicles are crushed or whose penis is cut off be admitted to the assembly of the Lord* and *The woman shall not wear that which pertaineth unto a man, neither shall a man put on a woman's garment for all that do are an abomination unto the Lord thy God.* Unfortunately, these examples of scripture show little understanding and tolerance for trans people but the quotes must be viewed in the same context as many other biblical views and opinions on minorities, which are in today's world viewed as outmoded rules and discriminatory. I use these quotes as a reference to illustrate the point that trans people are not a new entity and being misunderstood is a long-standing fact.

Molly Houses, which were a cross between a gay club and a brothel, existed in larger English cities in the

18th century. They were social venues where people could come to sing and dance and men could sit on each other's laps. Men were also allowed to dress in women's clothing and pretence weddings were also re-enacted as rituals amongst members. These were ideal outlets where trans people could go and express themselves without fear. Up until the 1960s it appears that clandestine options like this were the only viable means by which trans people could escape the emotional turmoil that resulted in them having to keep their true identity secret.

Trans people are coming more and more to the forefront of life in the Western world, but in other global cultures, though an established part of life, they face exclusion and separation in most instances. For example, in India the *hjiras* are male to female trans people who belong to a religious sect devoted to a particular goddess. Among many Native American groups there is a tradition of categorising such individuals as 'two-spirit' people – people with male bodies who identify and live as women, people with female bodies who identify and live as men, individuals of either sex who are sexually attracted to same sex others, or anyone who lives outside the traditional definitions of gender and combines elements of both female and male genders. Having two spirits is considered a special gift and some people are given special roles in religious ceremonies. In parts of Polynesia, a category called *mahu* incorporates males who adopt a female appearance and perform women's work.

Between the '50s and '70s, trans issues started to emerge in Western media when a small number of people who were publicly identified as having undergone gender reassignment surgery came to prominence. Since the 1970s we have seen hormone treatment and surgery becoming more readily available and the development of the internet has allowed trans people to explore their transition options more easily. The numbers of people coming out as trans is increasing quite rapidly and it is estimated that the number of gender nonconforming people who seek medical care is growing at 20 per cent per annum among adults and more than 50 per cent per annum among younger people.

David, trans man. 'During the '80s and '90s, trans people primarily went through the medical system and after genital reassignment surgery went back to living their lives. For many people, this was because they didn't want to be visible as trans people and preferred to go stealth. The disadvantage of this was that whilst they had corrected the physical aspect of their problem, their inward side received little emotional support to allow them to grow with confidence in their new lives. Although whilst things have changed for the better, different health authorities approach surgery differently, and often restrict the number of people it puts through surgery because of cost. This has led to more people travelling abroad to Thailand and Belgium for surgery. Many choose the latter because it is closer to home and whilst it is more expensive, family and friends have the option of visiting whilst they recuperate after surgery.'

Trans expression

There is no single authentic expression of trans identity. Trans people have a wide diversity of appearances, personal characteristics, interests, experiences and viewpoints. As mentioned earlier, trans includes trans men and women, non-binary people and cross-dressers, as well as people with a trans history that simply identifies them as men and women. In simple terms, this means it is impossible to give it a single definite meaning. There are many degrees of transition and options available to trans people and almost everyone chooses a unique personal pathway. Surgical status is not a reliable indicator as to how a person identifies, and therefore it is unwise to place those who have had surgery and those who have had little or no surgery, particularly genital reassignment, in different boxes. There are many trans people, regardless of identity, who do not have reassignment surgery for a variety of social and medical reasons, which I will expand upon later in the book.

Joan, trans woman. 'You have to conform more if you are trans because you have to make up for the past, for the time you lost whilst living a life that wasn't designed for you.'

Trans people have many different opinions about terminology, with some preferring medicalised terms and others preferring community terms. The term 'transsexual' was originally created as a psychiatric diagnostic label for people who seek medical assistance to transition permanently from male to female and from female to male. Therefore trans people who wished to receive medical approval for hormones or surgeries had no option but to accept being categorised as transsexual people. Increasingly, trans people are critical of the word 'transsexual' because they consider it can be an old fashioned pathologising term. However, some find it reassuring and legitimising to be medically referred to as being a transsexual person.

Katie, trans woman. 'There is this misconception, call it an urban myth, that I (and others like me) am a woman trapped in a man's body. I have not met any transsexual, myself included, who can completely relate to that. It was something the media latched on to 40 years ago to explain something they didn't understand. I can admit to feeling female and knowing that my male genitalia is wrong for me. This is an admission more commonly identified in the trans community.'

Libby, trans woman. 'I feel younger trans people respect the older ones. They know that things are different now – that things are easier. There is a terminology now that didn't exist 10–20 years ago. Making contact with other trans people and accessing support via the internet has never been easier. Young people often say to me, "Libby it must have been really hard. It's easy for us in comparison."'

With regard to what pronoun to use when speaking to or about a trans person, it is important to remember that a person's gender identity can differ from their appearance or the pitch of their voice. We should only use gendered pronouns such as 'he' or 'she' if we are certain that a person identifies themselves in that way. If we are not sure which pronoun to use, it is better to ask politely rather than make assumptions. It is equally advised to ask non-binary people what pronoun they prefer because some dislike being referred to as 'he' or 'she', preferring instead the more ambiguous pronouns of 'they' and 'them'. Cross-dressers like their persona to be referred to with a female pronoun when dressed in female clothing.

Robert, trans man. 'Cisgender people are privileged because their sex, chromosomes, hormones and secondary sex characteristics correlate with social understandings of what it means to be a man or a woman. They rarely ever have to think twice how they address somebody. Even people with the best intentions make mistakes from time to time. My advice is if someone pulls you up on gender identity listen to what they have to say and then afterwards address them as instructed.'

When considering how gender is viewed in society, it is primarily from a heterosexist perspective. Historically and culturally, we see men are expected to be masculine males who are strong, resilient and practical. We don't want to think of them as effeminate, queer, androgynous or weak. Women are expected to be feminine and it is generally expected that they be fragile, needy and maternal. We don't want to think of them as butch, aggressive or strong. In terms of dress codes, the Western world is prescriptive in how each gender is presented with certain colours, fabrics and clothing styles strongly gendered as masculine or feminine. Parents, teachers and peer groups exert pressure on children to conform to gender stereotypes. This forms a common root to transphobia and homophobia.

Why trans?

The role of biology is often a sensitive issue for trans people who prefer to use the description 'assigned at birth' when referring to their previous gender prior to transitioning, rather than 'biological sex'. The initial pathway to joining the category male or female begins at conception and thereafter through a series of developmental steps when a fertilised egg moves towards developing a body into a male or female foetus. Hilary Lips (2014) explains this process succinctly in her book, *Gender: The Basics*.

> When sperm meets egg to produce fertilisation, each normally contributes a set of 23 chromosomes, which pair up to form the genetic basis for the new individual. The 23rd pair, known as the sex chromosomes, is the pair that initially determines sex. Normally, this pair will be comprised of an X chromosome contributed by the mother's egg and either an X or Y chromosome contributed by the father's sperm. If the pair is XX, the pattern of development is predisposed to be female: if it is XY, the pattern is predisposed to be male. If some unusual combination, such as XO or XXX occurs, development tends to proceed in a female direction – as long as no Y chromosome is present. Only the sperm, not the egg, can contribute a Y chromosome. Thus the genetic basis of sex is determined by the father. (Lips 2014, p.6)

Nobody knows the precise reason why some people are trans. There is not yet any strong scientific evidence to explain atypical gender identity development. Having said that, it's estimated that autistic spectrum disorders occur at a higher rate in trans people than in the general population and that around 10 per cent of trans people, mainly trans men, are on the autistic spectrum. Research undertaken in 2011 by the University of Cambridge (Baron-Cohen and Jones 2011) found that trans men had elevated autism spectrum quotient scores compared with cisgender men and women and trans women. The research group hypothesised that trans men with more autistic traits may have had difficulty socialising with female peers and thus found it easier to identify with male peer groups. The research also hypothesised but did not entirely prove that trans men born with a higher level of male hormones were on the autistic spectrum.

Powerlessness is a prevalent feature of trans issues, primarily because research is generally limited, with governments dictating legislation and the psychiatric profession often relying entirely on opinions rather than facts. However, there has been some scientific research carried out on why trans brains do not correlate to their assigned male or female bodies. A study carried out by Zhou *et al.* (1995) at the Netherlands Institute for Brain Research, post-mortem on the brain materials of 43 human beings, concluded in their findings that in one area of the brain, male to female transsexual people have a typically female structure and female to male transsexuals have a typically male structure. Since then, a series of studies have associated brain differences with atypical gender identity development.

There is much speculation within the trans community itself as to why some people are transgender. Some of my interviewees came up with their own hypotheses.

Jayne, trans woman. 'There are several theories as to what makes a person feel in the wrong gender assigned to them at birth. It is a medical condition originating in the foetus. Certain hormones need to be at certain levels at various stages during pregnancy. There is the single twin syndrome. There is a theory from 30 years ago which suggested that if a woman was expecting twins – a boy and a girl – and that if one of them died either before or during birth, the remaining twin would want to take on the gender identity of their dead sibling. If it was a case of triplets and two of the babies survived, there would be 60 per cent of them wanting to be the gender of their dead sibling.'

Bianca, trans woman. 'No medical professional can tell you with certainty what causes someone to have dysphoria towards their assigned birth gender. They don't know whether it is caused by genetic factors or if something occurs during foetal development and growth of the brain. They don't know whether it is caused by factors pertaining to nature or nurture during childhood.'

Sherwin, trans man. 'Was my brain masculine in the womb from an early age? I wish there was medical research that held answers. I often wonder what biological basis there is to being trans. Is it caused by neurological factors or does something occur to a baby's hormones whilst in the womb? Personally, I intend to leave my brain to medical research to see if the scientists can come up with some answers.'

Natalie, trans woman. 'Why was I born trans? I'm not sure whether it was a fluke or not – just one of those things that happen. Was it a hormone imbalance in the womb? Was it something to do with brain development? Or maybe it is a genetic condition. The simple truth is nobody knows. All I know is that I have felt this way for as long as I can remember.'

Diversity and inclusion

Trans issues rarely receive prominence from governments across the Western world. Amnesty International, in their 2014 paper *The State Decides Who I Am*, summarises this point when referring to a person's identity and how people are officially recognised:

> Gender marker is a gendered designator that appears on an official document such as a passport or an identity card. It may be an explicit designation such as 'male' or 'female', a gendered title such as 'Mr' or 'Ms', a professional title, a gendered pronoun, or a numerical code which uses particular numbers for men and for women (for example – odd numbers and even numbers). (Amnesty International 2014, p.16)

Caroline, trans woman. 'Some people view trans as something that goes against the norms of society – and choose not to find out more about it and therefore never end up understanding it. We are viewed as having a medical condition. Yes, it is a mental condition. How can it not be? But it is not a mental illness. I am not mentally ill. Before I transitioned my brain and body did not match each other. I viewed it as something that was wrong with me that could be fixed. So I fixed it through years of treatments and surgeries. My journey is ongoing but I no longer see myself as somebody who has a problem any more.'

Trans people are in all walks of life, from university lecturers, pilots and computer scientists to nurses, teachers and secretaries. Like being gay, lesbian or bisexual, it could happen to anyone. It is something that can be found in any culture, race or social class. Although it has only crept into the public domain in the past 50 years, you will have already read it is something that has been around since the beginning of time. Therefore, it must be acknowledged that it probably exists in everybody's family ancestry, whereby millions of people will have died trans without ever publicly divulging this secret, through fear or shame.'

Andrew, trans man. 'Social standing has to be taken into consideration. Trans people will share various experiences according to economic and social backgrounds. Where you live, where you socialise and what you do for a living is also a factor. For many who use public transport daily, they too will have different experiences to share than those who travel everywhere by car. How you pass as a trans person is likewise true. The better you pass, the safer you are in public.'

Lili Elbe from Denmark was the first person to have had male to female reassignment surgery in 1930, as featured in *The Danish Girl* starring Eddie Redmayne. Michael Dillon was the first trans man to have full reassignment surgery (phalloplasty) in the UK, back in the 1940s. Originally from Folkestone in Kent, Dillon studied medicine at Trinity College in Dublin. In 1946, he published a book about transsexuality and this brought him into contact with Robert (who later became Roberta) Cowell (a racing driver and World War II fighter pilot), who was to later become the first trans woman in the UK to have reassignment surgery. This was no ordinary meeting as it led to Dillon performing an *orchidectomy* (removal of the testes) on Cowell before she later completed her reassignment surgery under another surgeon.

Other notable trans people include Christine Jorgensen who was an American GI who travelled to Denmark to have gender reassignment surgery in the early 1950s. She became the first highly publicised case, reported all over the world. Following her were Jan Morris, the travel writer, April Ashley; society model and restaurant hostess and Billy Tipton, the famous American jazz musician. Even to this day, all of these are still regarded as prominent figures when recounting earlier trans history.

Personalities who are becoming increasingly prominent in the media these days include Paris Lees, Kellie Maloney, Janet Mock, Caitlyn Jenner, Laverne Cox and Lana Wachowski, who is the producer, director and screenwriter of *The Matrix* film trilogy, *V for Vendetta* and *Cloud Atlas*. Then there is Thomas Beatie, who became famous when he got pregnant resulting in worldwide media interest in his pregnant body; Chaz Bono (son of the singer Cher); Jamison Green, who wrote *Becoming a Visible Man* and Riley Carter Millington, an actor in *Eastenders*.

Some trans people question if they should be part of the LGBT community. They feel the T part of this acronym is misplaced with some viewing themselves as a sub-group within the LGBT framework, whilst others feel they are outsiders within a community where they should feel protected and safe. There are many reasons why trans people were included in this framework alongside gay, lesbian and bisexual people – but mainly because it was felt that trans people were persecuted and had experienced similar societal discrimination as the gay community and hence a 'home' was created for them. However, not every trans person agrees with this assertion and feel the lines got blurred somewhere between sexual orientation and gender, with myths about gay men wanting to be women taken seriously and out of context, which has led to misinterpretation of what constituted a trans person.

Ruth, trans woman. 'I feel the T is just something that is tagged at the end of LGBT. Gay people can be as ignorant as anybody else in society about trans issues. They are equally capable of poking fun, making snide comments and sneering at us. These are hardly the actions of allies. Gay people need to educate themselves better by talking to trans people and listening to their life stories and experiences. It is only through this that they will begin to grasp what trans people are about and what their issues are, which will enable them to view life from a different perspective to theirs.'

Thomas, trans man. 'The T as part of LGBT has always been conflicted. Whilst it belongs within this framework, it doesn't always benefit. Many people in society confuse the issue and reflect upon it in terms of sexuality. But it is not a gay issue. Being trans is a process that is immensely different from being gay, lesbian or bisexual. Some trans people view it as a civil issue and feel it should not belong within a sexuality category with the other three groups. Others disagree, and refer to gay icons who do drag entertainment as champions to the cause. Whilst most drag queens and drag kings are not real trans people, they have nevertheless inadvertently brought into people's consciousness a degree of acceptance.'

Lifestyle choice?

There is no evidence to suggest that being trans is a lifestyle choice; in fact, if anything, biological science suggests the opposite. In the case of trans men and women – and non-binary people – much anguish is dealt with before the person comes to terms with their identity, and the idea that anybody would go through this as a matter of choice is difficult to imagine. As we have already seen in this chapter, trans people are experts on themselves because they have learned from each other in the absence of widespread medical expertise on the subject. Many healthcare providers know little about trans issues. There is hardly any trans awareness training among managers and staff, which makes it difficult for clients when they seek professional guidance.

Although society is changing, being trans is still seen as an eccentricity or a quirk that can be cured or changed. The battle against transphobia and discrimination continues and will be covered in a later chapter. There are feminist writers who espouse hatred towards trans women by claiming that only a cisgender female can genuinely feel what occupying a woman's body is like, for example through experiences such as having menstruation or childbirth. Trans men also get targeted and belittled by bigots who claim they are not being real men because they aren't able to produce sperm to father a child. The psychiatric profession believes it holds medical authority over trans people, although its investment into research is poor. Therefore, in the absence of scientific research that fully explains the condition, anecdotal evidence and personal experiences of trans people have to be heavily relied upon to explain to others how those who find themselves born with a brain that does not correlate with their body are faced with many challenges both internally and externally.

Iris, trans woman. 'The majority of trans people develop role models within their own communities. Many look towards the modern world and follow well-known trans people like Janet Mock in America and Lydia Foy in Ireland, who have fought for gender recognition for many years.'

Jeremy, trans man. 'Imagine a world where black and white people feel completely equal as each other with no hint of racial tension, and both peoples are completely at peace with one another and are able to live in harmony as a result. Trans people sometimes feel like black people who feel oppressed by white people. The main protagonist in the trans world is cisgender people. Legislation sounds excellent on paper but we are a minority group and the reality can be quite stark in terms of difficulties accessing healthcare and discrimination in employment, and there are many trans people who are disowned by their families in a way that gay people were 20 years ago. The trans world is backward in comparison to its lesbian and gay counterparts, but look how far the gay liberation movement has come along in the past 40 to 50 years since the Stonewall riots in America. The pattern of acceptance is slowly shifting in our favour. We are quickly catching up but must acknowledge that we are benefiting from the struggles of gay people who laid the foundation work in their quest for acceptance and equal rights.'

Psychiatric intervention

The World Professional Association of Transgender Health is best known by its acronym WPATH. Formerly known as the Benjamin Standards after Dr Harry Benjamin, an American psychiatrist who was a leading medical figure in the diagnostic criteria of transsexuals and an expert in transgender issues, WPATH is currently the official watchdog for standards of care for the health of transsexual, transgender and gender nonconforming people. In recent years it has moved from being a guidebook for gatekeepers to being an articulation of best care standards for the health and wellbeing of trans people. The organisation has a very good reputation across the Western world in trans communities because it has human rights at its core. It is considered a progressive organisation and an example of this is that it no longer excludes care for intersex people who are trans, something that was previously not given official recognition.

Unlike gay people, being trans is still considered a mental disorder in the psychiatric diagnostic manuals. There are two main internationally recognised psychiatric texts which are used to diagnose. The first of these is the World Health Organization's (WHO)

International Statistical Classification of Diseases and Health Related Problems (ICD-10) which defines gender identity disorder thus:

> A desire to live and be accepted as a member of the opposite sex, usually accompanied by a sense of discomfort with or inappropriateness of one's anatomic sex, and a wish to have surgery and hormonal treatment to make one's body as congruent as possible with one's preferred sex. (World Health Organization 2012, p.133)

The second and most commonly used text in the Western world is the *Diagnostic and Statistical Manual of Mental Disorder (DSM-5)*, which outlines the criteria required for a diagnosis of gender dysphoria (formally gender identity disorder). In general terms, this is defined in the manual as a condition where somebody experiences discomfort or distress because they feel their biological sex and gender identity do not match each other. In order to get a diagnosis of gender dysphoria, the manual specifies that two psychiatrists need to agree that a person fully demonstrates a marked incongruence between their experienced/expressed gender and the assigned gender at birth for a period of at least six months. Some of the factors that psychiatrists look for when making a diagnosis include determining if the client has a strong wish to be treated as the opposite gender (or an alternative gender, namely non-binary) they were assigned at birth, or if the person has a strong wish or longing to have the primary and/or secondary sex characteristics of the opposite gender they were assigned at birth. Other factors that are taken into consideration are if the client has a strong wish to get rid of their primary and/or secondary sex characteristics, or indeed if they have a strong wish to obtain the primary and/or secondary sex characteristics of the opposite gender they were assigned at birth. Psychiatrists can also diagnose gender dysphoria if the client believes and/or demonstrates that they already have typical feelings and reactions that are associated to the opposite gender they were assigned at birth.

Trans people need to have a diagnosis of gender dysphoria before they can be given hormone therapy or have reassignment surgery. Even if a person seeks private treatment, they still have to prove that they have been assessed by a psychiatrist and that they are of sound mind and in a position to give informed consent. This is not acceptable for some trans people who are becoming more and more critical of psychiatric labelling and mainly feel this is both unnecessary and demeaning. Progressive thinking, though, is spreading in the Western world. In 2010, France became the first country to remove trans identity from the list of mental diseases. Other countries are likely to follow in the years to come. The stigma of being labelled under the category of a mental disorder will be stripped away for ever.

Steven, trans man. 'We don't understand the brain. We don't understand emotions, thoughts and feelings and how these are structured within the brain. There are no tests available to psychiatrists and therefore anything that is not understood is placed into categories of mental disorder, which from the outset is stigmatising. Gender identity is something that is fluid, not rigid. Not every trans person will feel different from an early age. Many will have feelings of being different from early childhood but equally there will be others who will tell you that they were much older before they sensed difference.'

Intersex people

A question often asked is: where do intersex people fit within the trans community – or do they fit at all? Personally, I do not believe that they fit into this category in the conventional sense. Intersex people are born with sex characteristics that are inconsistent, for instance XY chromosomes and no penis or genitalia that are not easily identifiable as being male or female, or, more commonly, they may not be identified as having an intersex condition until they reach puberty and bodily changes do not take the usual course, or even later as adults, when a couple attends a fertility clinic because they are unable to conceive.

Mostly, those who discover they have an intersex condition at puberty or later will be content in their settled gender role, but just occasionally one of them might say: 'Ah – that explains how I feel', and will choose to transition. When a child is determined at birth to have an intersex condition, parents are often extremely distressed and they want a doctor to determine which gender they should use in raising their baby. In the past, some surgeons would alter the child's genitals to look more conventional. If a surgeon determines an intersex baby would be better converted to a female (as is often the case for convenience) and the baby's parents raise their *daughter* as a girl, but later on the child states *he* is male and chooses to transition, you have to wonder if transitioning would have been necessary had the surgeon not gone ahead and chosen the gender at birth. However, there are very few parents who agree to not have their child be given a gender label at birth.

Of course, that's a simplified rationale of a complex condition so let me explore it in more detail to outline the complexities. Intersex people may have chromosomal incongruities – XXY, XYY or YY – or some may have differences in their physical make-up (for example a woman may discover she cannot conceive because her ovaries are streaked with testicular material). Babies can be born with visibly ambiguous genitalia that does not entirely fit with what is considered male or female – for example a tiny penis but no testicles, or a large clitoris that resembles a penis, or a vagina instead of a penis but with testicles. There are over 40 known intersex variations. To the current day, it has been considered by many to be a shameful diagnosis that is rarely publicly divulged because of the fear and shame it evokes.

Diagnosis, up until recent years, led to corrective surgery at birth based on the surgeon's assumption about the baby's gender – followed by hormone therapy to match the assigned gender. Doctors often made errors of judgement which undoubtedly left many people in a distressed state by ending up having self-identified genders which did not match the gender to which their bodies had been surgically assigned. They may therefore decide to transition later in life. It is unknown how many intersex people transition because no studies have been done to determine numbers. However, it is important to know that being intersex is not the same as being trans, that the vast majority of trans people are not intersex and that the vast majority of intersex people are not trans.

Gary, intersex, trans man. 'As a female to male (FTM) trans intersexed person, I get thoughtless comments from non-intersexed trans people who say things like "You got the sex change I wanted." People fail to understand that I was mutilated at birth, which isn't actually anything like an adult sex reassignment. For a long time intersex people were not allowed to transition. The Benjamin Standards, which was the code by which doctors and therapists decided who could and could not be allowed to transition, specifically excluded intersexuals. This was because doctors who surgically assigned intersex babies at birth had to promise parents that the child would stay that way and not attempt to change gender later. The presence of trans people exposed that lie. That's why, when I transitioned 19 years ago, I had to lie about my intersex condition to get hormones.'

Now, many gatekeepers are no longer strictly following guidelines and intersex people are generally allowed to transition, although the issue of reassignment surgery is the same as that of trans people in the sense that sexual function and sensation after cosmetic genital surgeries is hit and miss. Endocrinologists get twitchy about giving us hormones. For many of us, our hormones are already not conventional for either men or women, and practitioners have to experiment with different dosages rather than just going with an ordinary dose step-up from the book. For example, I use only half the testosterone of a non-intersex FTM (I know because two of my partners are FTM), partly because my body already makes an intermediate amount, and partly because it is more sensitive to testosterone due to being intersex, so a little goes a long way.'

CHAPTER TWO

TRANSITIONING

Transitioning process

More and more people are transitioning now than ever before and the age at which they do so is lowering. Up until a few years ago, the majority of trans people were trans women who had been in their forties, fifties and sixties when they set out to transition to female. By that time, most were married and had children and sometimes grandchildren when they finally reached the decision that they could no longer live a lie and that the only way to escape from inner turmoil was to face the truth and seek help to live in the gender role that their brain always told was right for them.

There are three main hurdles to overcome in transitioning – social, medical and legal. The first step is the moment a trans person tells another person, be it a friend or family member, that their true gender identity differs from the gender they were assigned at birth.

Daniel, trans man. 'For some trans people who decide to transition, it enables them to make a fresh start from the past. They can leave their former lives, their former gender behind, and start afresh. But every human being is different and trans people share this uniqueness too in the sense that there will be those who accept personal responsibility for their past misdemeanours, and others who will justify their failings on their identity conflict. It is reasonable to assume that some will use it as a scapegoat for other failings in their life, thinking that they can bury all the bad things in their life when they transition. Often they are disappointed.'

Coming out as trans is a complex and challenging decision. It rarely comes without stress, anxiety and sleeplessness because of fear of being rejected, mocked or marginalised by others. Trans people often spend many years considering the risks of publicly changing their name, pronoun or gender presentation before they make any decision to do so. Even many years after gender reassignment trans people often still greatly fear that others who know their previous name and gender history may *out* them accidentally or deliberately. While many trans people do not look visibly trans, some have to deal with the ongoing frustration of being regularly outed by physical appearance or voice. Being gay isn't always visible whereas being trans is rarely invisible, at least in the early years of transition. Transphobia remains widespread and, although subtle at times, it can still shatter people's confidence.

Coming out as trans is a major step and careful preparation can smooth the process. However, sometimes people reach a sudden breaking point in regard to the stress of repressing such a core part of their identity. This may result in them blurting it out without any finesse or planning, increasing the risk of others failing to digest or understand the news in a favourable manner. However, even if the timing is not ideal trans people need to be free to come out on their own terms. It is offensive for other people to speculate publicly about whether someone might be trans, for example based upon their clothing, appearance or manner of speech.

Although attitudes towards trans people are improving, most trans people still end up facing some rejection from parents, family members, friends and colleagues. There may be elements of transphobia based on misinformation or ignorance. It is not unusual for people to resort to religion with some trans people telling me how they have encountered people who said to them, 'God will hate you, you need help – it is not normal what you're saying.' There will also be people who try to 'un-trans' the person by making unhelpful suggestions including seeing a therapist to avoid going through with transitioning. So a trans person needs allies to turn to for support and reassurance. Additionally, transitioning impacts on how others perceive the sexuality of the trans person and their sexual partner(s) so they may need support to deal with homophobia as well as transphobia. While non-trans friends can provide vital support, being able to speak to trans friends who have undergone similar experiences can be of particular benefit.

Once a person has decided to transition, the first step towards a referral needs to be made via their nearest Gender Identity Clinic (GIC) or Endocrinology Department (depending where in the Western world they live) and this is usually done by the person's general practitioner (GP) or by self-referral. Processes may vary in different countries so, for the purposes of simplicity, I will just describe what happens in the UK.

When the person is referred to the GIC they usually have to wait a minimum of six months before they are seen. Whilst they are on the waiting list to be seen they may change their name(s) if they haven't done so already and start dressing in their new gender. They may also decide to start some cosmetic surgical procedures including electrolysis and voice therapy.

After they are seen by their consultant, they will be prescribed hormone treatment but will need to live in their new gender role for 12 months to develop regular interaction with people. This period is also designed to try to ensure people have realistic expectations about what life will be like post-transition before they undergo irreversible surgery. After 12 months have passed and the trans person has received a diagnosis of gender dysphoria they will be referred for reassignment surgery, should that be their personal choice. Of course not every trans person wants to have surgery and even among those who do, there is variety in terms of which surgery or surgeries they want. For example, trans men often prioritise chest reconstruction surgery more than genital surgery.

Louise, trans woman. 'It's a process that each trans person has to follow rigorously. You have to obtain a diagnosis of gender dysphoria. To do so, you are asked to prove that you are trans by describing in detail what is it that makes you feel that your body and brain do not correlate to the same gender. The psyches want to establish that you are not a phoney, as well as proving that you are not some type of rebellious person who is out to defy society. After that you have to prove that you are compos mentis to have the treatment.'

Sarah, trans woman. 'My mind and psyche firmly believe I am female but my body is that of a male. While I am on the books at Charing Cross Gender Clinic waiting to be diagnosed with gender dysphoria, I am still hesitant about the transitioning process. I still believe I could go through with it but there are so many hurdles stopping me.

I am half Sarah – the woman I know I am. I am half David – the man I know I'm not. I go to work every day and present as David. In my mind, I am Sarah though, who sometimes pretends she is a man. All of my friends at work know about my gender dysphoria. My family, including my children and extended family, also know. I am a musician in my spare time and all my friends in the band know too.

At home, I am Sarah in every way. But as Sarah I rarely venture outdoors. The last time was two years ago when a lesbian friend almost dragged me out to a firework display. I needed much encouragement but she kept saying, "Let's do it, let's do it!" I relented and ended up having a very enjoyable time. Nobody paid the slightest attention to us. I was pleased that nobody mocked me. But I still lack the courage to repeat the experience.'

Isobel, trans woman. 'It's a matter of how a person approaches their medical practice. The first time I went to my GP, I guessed that she wouldn't know much about the subject so I printed off some NHS leaflets from the internet and took them along with me. My GP was honest and whilst thanking me for the printouts acknowledged that she knew little about the condition. In fact, we admitted that we were both learning together. She turned out to be a real ally and helped me in every aspect during my early days of transitioning, including my referral to the GIC and the prescribing of my hormone treatment once I had received a diagnosis of gender dysphoria.

I have heard horror stories about other trans people who went to their GPs and were quite demanding, stating they wanted this, that and the other and were affronted when their GPs weren't experts on the subject. Needless to say their overall experiences proved negative but they must be prepared to accept some level of responsibility in the way they approached the matter in the first place.'

Gender Identity Clinics (GICs)

Trans people must secure the approval of a psychiatrist at a GIC in order to access hormones and surgery to assist their transition. This gatekeeping creates a lot of fear and distress for many trans people, especially people with a non-binary gender identity who feel they may not be taken as seriously as trans men and trans women and fear being rejected and turned away.

Times are changing and trans people increasingly have the confidence to turn up in whatever they feel most comfortable wearing. However, this hasn't always been the case. GICs have in the past been renowned for expecting trans people to present in stereotypical clothing. It was at GICs that trans women were expected to present as ultra female and, up until recent years, deemed it necessary to turn up wearing a dress, long wig, stockings and high heels coupled with a handbag draped across their arm in order to be taken seriously as a woman.

Melissa, trans woman. 'A big worry for me before I started transitioning was: Will I pass? This was constantly on my mind. Thoughts of the proverbial pink dress and high heels continuously flashed across my mind, wondering if this really was the way I was expected to present outwardly for people to realise how I felt inside. This mindset had undoubtedly trickled its way down from the Gender Clinic where in the early days, at least, if a trans person did not make an effort to present almost stereotypically in their new gender role, they were not allowed to access services and were denied surgery. That meant trans women had to go all dolled with fake breasts, lots of rings and plastered in make-up and trans men were expected to wear lumber jackets, check shirts and boots. But these days the Clinic makes a point of saying to everyone that they must not feel pressurised to dress in any particular way and hence the farce of this pretence dressing is becoming history.'

George, trans man. 'You have 15 minutes to sell yourself as a trans person so the way you dress is important. For trans men, they look for a short back and sides style haircut. The doctors are looking for what they consider the typical story: someone telling them that they have felt the opposite gender to birth since the age of three or four. They want you to make sure that you are making the correct decision and place great emphasis on how people must live openly as a trans person. They tell you how hormone therapy will affect your life and how reversal is difficult or impossible based on how far you take the transition process. But what's not taken into consideration is coming out to family and friends – the impact of this, the lack of support that is sometimes available and how the stress of this is just as irreversible as anything else in the transition process.'

There are long waiting lists at GIC because the number of trans people seeking treatment has increased greatly, especially in the last ten years. In the UK the service is slowly expanding to accommodate the increase in referrals but it is still not unusual for a trans person to be on a waiting list between 12 and 36 months before they are seen. There are some differing views on favouritism within the system with some trans people being more patient than others.

Hannah, trans woman. 'Young people need to exercise patience. I waited until my early sixties to start transitioning. I say to young trans people who are in their twenties and thirties, who complain about waiting lists at the Gender Clinic, that their lives don't have to come to a standstill while they're waiting. There is so much to learn and discover about your new life while you are waiting.'

John, trans man. 'The tide is definitely turning at GICs, because more trans people now exist than at any other time in history, simply because people now know how easy it is to transition. How trans people are perceived is changing, thus making it more acceptable and more comfortable to engage in the process. Years of putting up and shutting up are gone. People like myself no longer have to put up with being a masculine woman. The chance to rethink is upon us. The longing to be male instead of female is no longer a dream, rather something more and more people are turning into reality.'

Diana, trans woman. 'I personally feel that Gender Clinics are ageist and that if you are a younger trans person you will go through the system quicker. I know friends who have waited years to be referred on for reassignment surgery and have been kept waiting – whilst younger people who arrived after them seem to have jumped the queue a bit faster.'

For some people an indefinite wait leads to increased anxiety levels and depression. Research carried out by the Scottish Transgender Alliance, which carried out an online survey of over 800 trans people in 2012, found an overwhelming dissatisfaction from its participants about the service they receive or had received from their Gender Identity Clinics (McNeil *et al.* 2012). The overall picture indicated that, despite some people encountering friendly medical professionals, the service itself lacked a sense of organisation and competence. The following is an example of the opinions expressed which is indicative of the tone of several others. Names and gender were not used in the feedback results:

I experience the NHS GIC service as largely a paternalistic gatekeeping exercise where psychiatrists exercise inappropriate levels of control over the lives and choices of patients. They ensure compliance by withholding or threatening to withhold access to treatment (hormones, surgery). Their primary purpose seems to be to make it as difficult as possible for people to access the hormones/surgery they need in order to save the NHS money.

There is no transparency about the treatment pathway or clinical protocols, which leads to a Kafkaesque situation where clinicians are making decisions that directly affect your life, but you have no knowledge or say about how those decisions are being reached. There are a few good, compassionate clinicians working in the GICs but they are the exception in the system that is set up to maintain the paternalistic control of a few egotistical psychiatrists over their patients.

Having to negotiate the GIC system seriously hindered my transition. At many times, it has left me feeling angry, disappointed, manipulated, controlled and despairing. The system is deeply flawed. (McNeil *et al.* 2012)

Hormone treatment

The aim of hormone therapy for trans people is to alleviate the psychological distress of not being comfortable with their appearance as a man or as a woman, and who are in conflict with the gender into which they were assigned at birth. The physical effects, for example, on libido or fat distribution of the hormones naturally produced by the testes in trans women (testosterone) and ovaries in trans men (oestrogen), may also be unwelcome. Therefore, one of the first major steps in bringing relief to this inner turmoil, which many trans people have experienced since a young age, is to start hormone therapy to counteract the effects of their naturally occurring hormones and help them to become more feminine or masculine in their appearance.

Elaine, trans woman. 'I have taken Progynova – a type of oestrogen – for the past five years. My psychiatrist recommends this as it is good at preventing baldness as well as prostate cancer. I have also had electrolysis and laser surgery to control growth of facial hair. The rest of my body is hairless.'

Hailey, trans woman. 'It's not a problem for me being on hormone treatment for life. I'm used to it now after 15 years. Besides, I've had reassignment surgery, so in the absence of testes my testosterone is almost non-existent. These days I wear oestrogen patches twice weekly which are like those worn by menopausal women who undergo HRT treatment. I don't experience side-effects but do occasionally have days when I feel anxious, but this only lasts for a day or two.'

Changes usually start to take place after a few months and once established they may be difficult to reverse. For trans women taking oestrogen, fat may be distributed on the hips. The penis and testicles will reduce in size. Erections and orgasms become harder to achieve. Breasts begin to grow. The growth of facial and body hair becomes considerably weaker, although there might still be a need for electrolysis. The development of baldness will be slowed down. For trans men taking testosterone, this will enable facial and body hair to grow, although some may go bald. Testosterone helps develop a deepening of the voice. The clitoris gets bigger and will start getting erections. Libido is heightened, muscle bulk increases and periods stop.

Some trans people report significant differences to their emotional wellbeing and mental health as a result of taking hormones. However, there seems to be a marked difference in outcome between those taking masculinising hormones and those on feminising hormones. In the main, trans men on masculinising hormones find that they experience some degree of emotional dampening, short temperedness and generally find it more difficult to cry. They also report dramatic increases in energy, stamina and libido. In contrast, trans women on feminising hormones generally describe feeling calmer, more emotionally expressive and more sensitive to their surroundings, making them more prone to crying. Some also experience a decrease in energy and libido.

Some trans people experience mood swings when starting hormone treatment and some endure increased problems with memory and concentration. This is believed to be a result of the chemical changes produced by the hormones and the emotional responses to the physical changes that the hormones induce. In other words, trans people are likely to experience a combination of the direct effects of the hormone itself as well as the greatly welcomed physical changes that the hormones bring to their bodies. This, in turn, affects the way they interact with the world and, consequently, how they are seen and treated by society, which again affects their emotional wellbeing. However, it is considered that the vast majority of trans people who undertake hormone therapy are satisfied with their bodies and their emotional wellbeing as a result of this.

Surgery

Hundreds of thousands of people in the Western world attend Gender Identity Clinics each year to seek change from their assigned gender at birth. Funding for surgery through the various health authorities in most European countries is a contentious issue with some authorities allowing it more freely than others, prompting some trans people to travel overseas and privately fund their surgery instead. It is worth noting that private medical insurance does not provide for this kind of elective surgery. The main barrier for surgery in public health services is that it is considered too costly to fund and they regard it as elective and sometimes unnecessary. In the UK, trans people are legally entitled to treatment on the NHS but may also choose to be treated privately. The difference between public health services and private treatments is paramount. If your income is low or you are unemployed, trans people have to rely on the former, which undoubtedly entails long waiting lists and requires patience. If trans people have a good level of disposable income, private treatment brings many advantages.

Trans people may decide to have different types of reassignment surgery. For trans women, this consists of breast construction which may be followed by genital surgery which can include the removal of testicles (orchidectomy) and/or followed by a vaginoplasty (creation of a vagina).

For trans men, the key non-genital surgery is chest reconstruction by removing the breasts. This can then be followed by a hysterectomy to remove the ovaries and uterus and/or followed by phalloplasty (creation of a penis) or metoidioplasty (enlarging the clitoris into a small penis).

As mentioned earlier, a trans person needs to have lived full time in their new gender role for one year before being offered genital surgery. Despite long waiting lists and complex procedures, surgery is still the wish of many trans people. Although there have been constant improvements in surgical procedures, and the results can now be aesthetically pleasing, it is known that new genitalia does not always work as well sexually as natural born organs, often leaving the person feeling disappointed and demoralised.

Jacinta, trans woman. 'Everybody experiences body dysphoria differently. What makes a person happy is individual to them, hence it is wrong to inflict surgery upon those who do not want it. The way that certain societies think about trans people needs to change. To achieve this, the first step is to depathologise the psychiatric diagnosis. It is not a mental illness or disorder. It is a complex situation. The mind, body and spirit can go through a transition and needs to be reconciled. A counsellor may help untangle this complexity to bring about unity in this inner torment and self-loathing.'

Anthony, trans man. 'Make sure you are ready for every step. Don't be pushed into anything you don't want to do. Before you are ready for transitioning, you must have reached a high degree of comfort with yourself. Only you can say what you feel comfortable about. This entails finding your level of comfort and staying with that. You don't have to copy or keep up with somebody else. You don't have to take hormones unless you want to and you don't have to borrow money to have surgery, unless that's what you really want to do. You must listen to yourself in order to get it right. Transitioning is different for everyone. Nobody knows how others feel or think. Nobody can tell you what it feels like to be a man but you.'

Legal recognition

Different countries have different rules regarding when a trans person can have their self-identified gender legally recognised. Many countries in Europe still have onerous requirements that undermine trans people's human rights and dignity, requiring trans people to undergo removal of reproductive organs (resulting in irreversible sterilisation) before legal documents are changed to reflect their new gender. Others do not have any clear procedures for changing legal gender, whilst several require compulsory divorce of any partner before granting gender recognition.

The UK Gender Recognition Act 2004 allows trans people who have lived permanently in their new gender role for a minimum period of two years to apply for a Gender Recognition Certificate (GRC). There is no requirement for genital surgery or indeed any other medical treatment before the issue of a GRC. Once this document is issued, people may, if their birth was registered in the UK, use it to apply for a new birth certificate in their new gender and name. The two year wait was put in place after those responsible for drafting the Act asked the passport office if and when trans people who had changed their passports asked to change them back. The passport office confirmed that if trans people realised that transition was a mistake and asked for their passport to be restored to their old name and gender, it was almost always within the first two years of their transition. It has been argued that this is simply an appropriate safety net, designed to ensure that people do not change their legal gender too quickly, finding themselves then trapped into a way of being that they realise is not right for them.

In the UK, at the time of transition a trans person can, however, change their name and gender on almost all of their legal documents, including their driving licence, passport, bank account, employment and medical records. They can do this by providing proof of name and gender change, normally a statutory declaration notarised by a solicitor or clerk of the court. The declaration details their old name and gender and their new name and gender, and their intention to use them permanently from the date of signing. These are all concessions made by the British government over the last few decades after campaigning by trans activists. However, despite this the applicants are still of their legal gender until they have obtained formal gender recognition.

Trans men and women may then marry or enter into civil partnership in that gender status and name. If they are already married or in a civil partnership, they are issued an Interim GRC, which they must use to annul that relationship before being issued with the GRC, after which they qualify for a new birth certificate. Alternatively, they may convert their marriage into a same sex marriage or their civil partnership into a marriage, but only if their spouse agrees. The Gender Recognition Act does not permit non-binary or non-gender status to be recorded on a birth certificate.

Intersex people may obtain an amended birth certificate without using the Gender Recognition Act if their condition was noted at, or soon after, birth. Nonetheless, some intersex people who have transitioned later may be able to use the Act to obtain a new birth certificate, because they may undergo the same process as trans people in order to access treatment. Doctors do not include information about their intersex condition in their application documents.

There is a handful of Western world countries who have become more progressive by allowing self-declaration for all transgender people so that a trans person is automatically believed about their preferred gender. This means trans people living in these countries do not have to undergo any psychiatric evaluation, or be obliged to live in their new gender role for a period of time, or have surgery before they were officially able to change their legal documentation.

Harry, trans man. 'Some parts of the world are making progress; take, for example, Argentina, Denmark, Ireland and Malta where there are better laws for trans people coupled with societal acceptance. These countries have striven to implement legislation that incorporates self-determination whereby a transgender person is taken at his or her word and can gain legal recognition without seeing a doctor.'

Role of the internet

The internet's role in encouraging dialogue within the trans community has gathered momentum in every aspect. Support is at the end of anyone's fingertips. There are ample websites and forums that facilitate discussion and help is readily available to people who are still coming to terms with their identity and in need of help and guidance. But the advice for using the internet to access information comes with the same warning as it does on most other issues, and that is to take care. Here are some views expressed by my interviewees.

Olivia, trans woman. 'The internet is able to distort or enhance any subject but is, on balance, good. I think the trans community would be lost without it but it needs to be used with caution. There is a lot of very good and sound information available if you know where to look for it. There are several websites that offer support and advice for people who are initially too nervous or scared to talk to their doctor about transitioning. This allows them to get in touch with other like-minded people for peer support and guidance. A person can learn from peers about where to go locally for help. There are websites which inform trans people about the best places for chest reconstruction, as well as reassignment surgeries. I personally have found the internet useful for information and tips on clothes, feminising my behaviour and support regarding personal safety. There are also plenty of YouTube clips too, which show make-up demonstrations as well as short films of trans people sharing some of their life experiences, along with general tips for coming out and transitioning.'

Gerald, trans man. 'The internet is capable of misleading people. If you search "trans" on a search engine, you will come up with about 70,000 entries and a high percentage of these will not be very good. In fact, some will be exaggerated rubbish. It is simply a matter of what the person is looking for. Remember this is information from all over the world that may not apply to you – or where you live. There are some trans people who only read what they want to read and don't check out who wrote it or check into the validity of what's written. In the case of buying hormone treatment online, some people expect overnight changes and often end up disappointed with the results that they interpret as not being as good as promised. They then double the dosage which can have serious consequences. If sex and pornography is what you want, you will find plenty but again much of this is liable to be misleading. It is suspected that some of the trans women are biological women pretending to be trans. Others look beautiful on screen but you have got to be sceptical and wonder what some of them would look like if you met them walking down the street. Cyber sex works for some people and helps them to release frustrated feelings whilst masturbating to images. Chat rooms are good places to go for companionship provided you don't get forced into saying or agreeing to anything you're not comfortable with.'

CHAPTER THREE

MALE TO FEMALE (MTF)

Valerie. 'Twenty years ago, I would have objected to being called a man. Today, I couldn't care less. I have had full reassignment surgery and feel like a woman in every way possible. Now I am comfortable in my own skin and am oblivious to other people's misconceptions and biases.'

There is no standard way of describing what it is like to be a trans woman in today's world because there is no neat single description that fits all, except for one common denominator: all trans women believe they were assigned the wrong gender at birth. They self-identify as female despite being assigned as male at birth. How they choose to express their gender identity varies considerably, although most trans women do use hormone therapy when transitioning to live in a feminine role.

The following two interview extracts feature Liz, who at the time of our interview was still tentatively working out her identity and considering her options, and Alice, who had completed her transition.

Liz. 'I secretly dressed in women's clothes behind my wife's back throughout our marriage. By the time I told her my secret, which signalled the end of my marriage, I had quite a stash of clothes hidden in the loft, along with my high heels and make-up. When my wife went out for evenings with her friends, I would dress up and have a lovely relaxing few hours. And what bliss it was when she went away for weekends to see her elderly parents, and then I was able to be Liz – the real me – for an entire weekend without fear of interruption, as we lived in a rural area. However, the dread of answering the door to the postman without thinking beforehand of how I was dressed, was ever present. I'm not sure what he might have thought had I done that!

I sometimes worry – and I know one of my sons certainly does too – that people will think I am a cross-dresser who dresses in women's clothing for some kind of sexual fetish. I hope I am not sounding discriminatory here. I know I may even show some ignorance, but cross-dressers don't always get good press. My son has requested that he never sees me dressed as Liz. "Dad, I know what you are, but we need to have you in our lives as you are and not someone else." The irony is he has only ever known me as someone else. It is Liz that is the real me. My other son and daughter don't have a problem with it. In fact my daughter, who by social norms should be most upset because she was, when younger, a "daddy's girl" has proved to be the most relaxed of them all. She has told me that when her children are older that she is going to introduce me to them as Liz, as this is the person she would most like them to get to know.

I'm considering all my options. I have talked to a support group over the telephone and have been invited to go and meet with them in person. I am at a crossroads really and know that if I am to be ever truly happy, I need to be brave and make some kind of formal announcement to signal the end of my old life – the part of me that has never been ME: a shadow – a life continuously built on lie after lie. There don't have to be any more lies now. My children know my secret and I know that is probably the hardest bit over as far as telling close family is concerned. But I fear transitioning is like taking a leap into the unknown. But it is a leap that is necessary to take, if I am to become the person I have always been in my mind.'

Alice. 'I knew there was something wrong around the age of eight or nine, but when you're young, you haven't got the skills to analyse things. I used to look at my sisters and feel they were so lucky. The more I thought about this, the more my fantasy formed that I would like to be a girl. But for now, I was stuck. I wasn't comfortable playing football but I wasn't allowed to do anything the girls did like dressmaking. To make matters worse, my parents sent me to an all-boys grammar school when I was 13. I made up my mind on the first day that I hated being a boy and hated being surrounded by boys. I thought more and more about being a girl. I thought there was something wrong with me, that I must be mad. My grandmother had dementia and for some reason was put in a mental hospital. I remember visiting her with my mother and thinking how it resembled a prison with bars on the windows. I genuinely thought, "How can I ever tell anybody that I want to become a girl? If I do they will incarcerate me like my grandmother." There was nobody to turn to in those days. Nobody would have known what was going on in my mind anyway, and nobody would have heard the word "trans". So my secret remained firmly guarded.

In my late teens, I decided I had to snap out of it. I decided that if I got a girlfriend, then I would be a man. She was a little older than me and had a little boy who I loved. After we got married I adopted him. We went on to have two girls. It felt like domestic bliss. I loved looking after the children, which was good because their mother was lazy and did little to help raise them. I didn't mind because I loved being their "mother". I washed, played and fed them, helped with their homework and put them to bed. In hindsight, I was a good mother but a lousy husband. I paid little attention to my wife, although we never argued. Eventually, the marriage foundered and she met someone else. In those days, the mother automatically got custody of the children. I still saw them at weekends but my life was turned upside down in just a few weeks. I became very depressed because the children were my life. It was interesting to note years later, however, that the bond I created with them as young children remains to this day; they are much closer to me than their mother.

Aged 26, with a broken marriage and limited contact with my children, I was rendered completely depressed. The thoughts of wanting to be a woman returned. It had never occurred to me to dress up as a woman when I was married, but I know that in order to suppress these feelings I threw myself into work. I got an accountancy apprenticeship and went to college a few days each week. I kept busy. My parents were really proud when I was promoted but my thoughts were still dominated with being a woman. Then I thought of the last remedy that had worked and got another girlfriend. I was 31 and she was ten years younger. We had two boys together. Domestic bliss returned. My second wife was a much better mother than my first. We were more compatible and went out for meals and to the cinema. Whenever she went shopping for new clothes, I used to join her as she valued my opinion. I genuinely loved her and was deeply upset that history repeated itself and we divorced. I was 51; back to square one and the thoughts re-emerged.

Then the internet was born and I began my research. I remember saying to myself, Oh my God, it's called transgender! There was a name for the real me and for the first time I realised that my life could change. I started dressing as a woman to see what it felt like and discovered the difference between happiness and contentment. Let me explain. Whilst I was happy looking after the children and satisfied with my job and its perks, there was always something missing, a discontentment that I didn't realise until I began transitioning and it was then that a deep sense of peace, serenity and fulfilment filled a deep void.

All but one of my five children are fine with me as a woman. My eldest son was in the RAF when I first started transitioning and for a while could not bring himself to speak to me. But I kept in touch and always sent Christmas and birthday cards. When he left the RAF he started a new relationship and his girlfriend coaxed him round. According to my other children, she said, "What are you worried about? This could happen to anyone." So afterwards he got back in touch by text messages and emails. Although he still struggles and isn't ready to meet up, he appears to understand. I know we will meet up eventually but only when he's ready. My other children call me by my first name in public, although in private I'm Dad. I am close to my grandchildren too, who are growing up and know me as Alice.

I feel totally content these days because now I am the real me. When I moved to Scotland to make a fresh start, I decided I was ready to have surgery. Afterwards, I felt I was fully a woman. It's the simple things that make an enormous difference, like being able to wear a proper bathing costume when I go swimming without worrying about being stared at every time. Before surgery, I was ashamed of hiding my male genitalia. It didn't feel right that I had breasts but also a penis and testicles. For me, there's no point in half measures. I wanted to be totally a woman and now I am, both physically and mentally.'

The overwhelming response from trans women is that the majority of them stated that they can remember thinking from early childhood that there was something different about them. However, this incongruence only troubled them when they were compelled to act differently – for example, when told not to play with girls or asked to do something they were uncomfortable with such as playing a sport in which they had no interest. In the absence of pressures from family, friends and society to be different, they felt happy and content within themselves. When conformity against their natural selves was impressed upon them, this became problematic and doubly so when this meant having to go against what they considered to be natural, normal behaviour – which, in essence, it was.

Stephanie. 'I was trapped in a male-built body but from the age of three I knew that this did not match my brain. To explain this in simple terms, I was a woman who was physically developing as a male but I had a female brain that controlled my thoughts and feelings. I remember being in a ballet at infant school and wanting to wear a tutu because it seemed the most natural thing for me to wear, but my mother sternly told me that I must wear a leotard like the rest of the boys – but I knew even then that she was wrong and I was right. Although I grew up knowing that I was not like everyone else, I learned to act like people expected me to act.'

In order to be accepted by others and to blend into society, some trans women will have gone to extraordinary lengths prior to their transitioning. Referred to as the flight into hyper-masculinity, this can entail anything from growing a beard in order to look as masculine as possible, or going to the gym to participate in pursuits that are viewed as strong and macho. It is primarily prompted by an inner conflict within the person. Those concerned feel that external factors can somehow change the thoughts they are having of being a woman by somehow convincing their brain that they are male. Getting married is another factor that some think will reverse how they feel about themselves, but they soon discover that this too fails to work.

Claudia. 'I hated the way I felt and did my best to live up to a macho image. I felt if I could manage this, the feelings would go away and I would feel peace from my inner torment, so I grew a beard. I loathed myself every time I looked in the mirror. My self-confidence couldn't have been lower so I shaved the damn thing off. Afterwards, I got out my compact set, did my make-up and felt instant relief.'

Fathering children is another unsuccessful attempt to reverse gender dysphoria. It, too, becomes part of denial and internalised transphobia, that is, hatred towards the self. These actions are often carried out because they are perceived as necessary to conform to society. But they never break the feelings of wanting to be a woman, nor do they alleviate unhappiness, depression or low self-esteem. My interviewees made it quite clear that acceptance is the only escape route out of this dilemma. It is only then that they realise they can no longer hide their real identity and, in doing so, they finally start feeling normal and natural for the first time in their lives.

Trans women recognise that many non-trans people feel awkward around them and are unsure how to treat them. They know there are those that believe it is a lifestyle choice. They have heard all the innuendos that circulate in society about them – man in a frock, she-man, oops he's had a sex op! But they continue with their transitioning because they know it is the correct thing to do. They also know there is no turning back into somebody they never were in the first place.

Anne. 'You sweat, sometimes you feel as if you are wringing wet. Even when I went out in low-heeled shoes, I didn't want to be recognised. But that's all right. It's not like I was out robbing or killing people.'

The following four extracts from Leona, Fleur, Judith and Poppy highlight the feelings of incongruence experienced from an early age and show self-acceptance once the women realised what they needed to do to live comfortably in their true gender role. In general, these women enjoyed positive experiences from family members, which was an important factor in building their self-confidence, especially when they came out initially and emotions were raw with them fearing everyone and worrying that everything may turn against them.

Leona. 'I was envious of my sisters when I was young. I wanted to dress like them. I was envious of girls in my class at primary school. I too wanted to wear ribbons in my hair like them. When I was four I was upstairs at home and slipped into one of my sister's petticoats, when suddenly I heard my father coming up the stairs. I quickly hid. I froze with fear, dreading that he might catch glimpse of me. Luckily he didn't. Here I was at this young age expressing myself how I wanted to be, how I should be, but when I recounted this story to my psychiatrist he pointed out to me that my dysphoria had started at a young age because I instinctively knew that it was taboo to have dressed in my sister's underclothes. But there was a part of my brain that didn't want me to reveal myself because it protected me from the shame I would have felt if my father had caught me. It was the start of the biggest secret I have ever kept in my life.'

Fleur. 'The fact of the matter is pretty simple. My brain doesn't allow me to think or live as a man. I have always been a female but once I stopped resisting my inner feelings and started listening to my heart, there was no turning back. My strict Catholic upbringing had inserted a little voice in the back of my head that told me dressing as a woman was something that men weren't supposed to do. I was made to think it was something that social outcasts and perverts did. Even at 38, I still struggled internally and decided to seek counselling but, after a full year in therapy, I still could not settle for a life which didn't allow me to express my femininity. I joined the trans scene and made more sense of my life than I ever did during counselling. It made me realise that there was a woman inside of me, not a man, and this was what I had been yearning to express all my life.

Although, I had never been in a relationship, sexuality wasn't an issue. Back then, I would clearly have identified myself as heterosexual – there was even a woman I loved from a distance. But my new self-perception made me realise that I didn't want to be with her, I wanted to be her. I knew that I was jealous of her and the other women who had the freedom to express themselves without being judged. I realised that I got along better with women on hormone treatment and planning reassignment surgery than those who cross-dressed. I knew this was the route for me.

I started hormone replacement therapy around the same time as I told my family. They were understanding, or at least as accommodating as they could be within the confines of society. Oestrogen became the food for my brain. I remember one of the first times I ventured out walking by myself. It felt so natural and so real that I never wanted it to end. I broke down and cried because I had never felt so alive before. It was pure ecstasy.'

Judith. 'We were a conservative family but my father stood out as someone with liberal views. Considering it was only the 1970s, his views were progressive for the era. He had a warm nature and there was nothing I couldn't divulge to him. When I was 17, I told him I was a girl, born into the wrong body. I still remember him gently closing his eyes and saying, "Stick with it, it will pass." But it didn't and I did everything in my power to make it pass.

Time was not rationed either because after that conversation I spent the next 27 years trying everything to avoid becoming the person I had been all my life – including marriage and children. Then I reached a point where I could no longer tolerate living a lie. That is not to say that I used my ex-wife as an excuse in the process. I loved her and still do, so she was not deceived in that sense. Simply, the time came when I had to do something about the way I was feeling inside. The woman within had to be freed.'

Poppy. 'As a young child, I was confused about clothes and toys. I couldn't understand why I wasn't allowed to wear dresses or play with dolls. It seemed so unfair. Even at a young age, I forced myself to snap out of it and tried to fit in. In my early teens, I became more individual and more ambitious. I organised dressing up games with my older sisters and their friends and I always played the damsel in distress. I loved wearing pearls, a dress and shoes and loved the humour associated with the game. In my late teens, I entered the inquisitive stage and started dressing in my bedroom. I would stand in front of the mirror in my older sister's clothes, feeling sexier than I had ever felt before. For the first time in my life, I liked my reflection. I saw a beautiful young woman who was me. At last I was true to myself.

I became so impatient with my parents and sisters and couldn't wait for them to go out at weekends. I had bought a new collection of skirts and blouses and wanted to model them around the house without fear of being interrupted. Thank God for make-up. It covers a multitude of sins. I have continuously worn ladies' underwear since the age of 19. It was the one thing that kept me sane before I came out, that little bit of me that felt whole. Later on, I became clever and bought androgynous clothing as much as possible. I chose garments that I considered nobody would recognise the difference. Gay people have it so much easier than trans people. No matter how closeted they are, they can dress as they like and look as they want without this added pressure.

When I told my parents, they were absolutely fine and when they told me that they still loved me I burst into tears. This gave me the confidence to start buying my own clothes and I felt I looked more like a woman with every day that passed. There was one day though when I was out shopping with my mother that I felt a dip in my confidence. I remember saying, "Mum please come with me", but she was preoccupied looking at something and I had no sooner started walking towards the toilet door when I heard, "There's a bloke going into the female toilet." But to my delight, my mother piped up, "No, that's my daughter, leave her alone."'

Passing

In general, not all trans women get along with each other. Why would they? Likewise for all trans people, because they are exactly the same as everybody else in any community where there is tension, expectations and sometimes unkindness. I think it is necessary to highlight this point, rather than to paint a picture of a perfect utopia. However, despite this, it is also important to point out that there appear to be more allies within the trans community, and indeed the larger LGBT community, than there are adversaries. Support groups are still an important asset to trans women who can meet like-minded people for informal guidance, advice and support. Lasting friendships are usually formed here.

Trans women worry perhaps more than other trans people about how they present to the world. Sex identities within society result in women having their appearance scrutinised and criticised far more harshly than men. Additionally, women's experiences of oppression from men results in greater hostility towards visibly trans women entering female single sex spaces than visibly trans men face entering male single sex spaces. This places trans women under great pressure to fulfil societal stereotypes of femininity if they wish to avoid being perceived as trans and subjected to transphobic comments about their appearance.

Fiona. 'Passing is an obsession to other trans women. They constantly fret about how well they look in their new gender, and wonder if they can go about their daily lives without fearing that everyone knows they have transitioned. It's what they talk constantly about to their friends. They compare themselves to their friends and things can get very bitchy on the trans scene if one woman passes better than someone else. Jealously and bitchiness is not uncommon. Indeed, some women pass better than others. Less practice means that they may not have developed a good sense of clothes style and make-up. Some are large-shaped whilst others are naturally petite. Some have spent a lot of money on surgery, for example they may have had their Adam's apple removed. Breast enhancement or facial electrolysis may have worked better for them than it did for others. But what is crucial to all of this is confidence, rather than how you look. It's how you feel about yourself that matters and not how others see you from the outside. Some trans people are very kind-hearted and will take newer ones under their guidance. Others will be jealous and bitchy, particularly if you are young and look good.

There is also envy towards those who come out and go through their transition quickly, particularly those who know what they want and don't hesitate in having surgery. If you are one of those people and you have a successful career and a good social life, expect resentment.'

The rights of trans women have gathered increasing support in the past decade because, every year, more and more choose to transition. With greater media attention and generally more empathetic coverage as a whole, society is slowly but surely edging closer towards wider acceptance. This is not to imply that being a trans woman is easy in today's world, rather that it is becoming easier – but high levels of ignorance and transphobia still prevail, which I will address later in the book. If the current trend towards wider acceptance continues to evolve at a steady pace, it is envisaged that the day will arrive when society embraces trans people with the same level of respect that gay people now receive.

Antonia. 'Up until about ten years ago, people did not express their trans feelings until much later in life, whereas these days people are transitioning much younger. To a certain degree, I sought comfort in late teens and throughout my twenties by being a Goth, where it is acceptable to wear make-up and nail varnish and to dress in ambiguous clothing. I was 30 when I began hormone therapy. Some young people these days are fortunate enough to have the option of taking puberty blockers. In the case of young trans women in these circumstances, they develop better bone structure earlier in life with the blockers. Better information and a better general awareness of trans issues in young people are allowing them to express their feelings earlier in life. Maybe society is more open-minded than we think.'

Surgery
Trans women may decide to have different types of reassignment surgery. Non-genital surgeries can usually

take place at any point in someone's transition. In addition to breast and genital reconstruction surgeries, there are various other procedures trans women can undergo, including surgery to chin, forehead and face and surgery to make the Adam's apple less prominent. Many hours of electrolysis are required to rid the face of facial hair and prevent beard growth, and hair transplantation may be required to undo male baldness. Every trans woman dreads a shaving shadow appearing underneath their make-up.

In contrast to non-genital surgeries, genital surgeries are usually only permitted after at least 12 months living full-time in the new gender role. For trans women, the most commonly undergone genital surgery is vaginoplasty (using the skin of the penis to construct the vagina and the tip of the penis to construct the clitoris). However there are also other vaginoplasty techniques, using different tissues, and also some trans women may decide to undergo orchidectomy without any vaginoplasty. As previously mentioned, some trans women do not undergo any genital surgery as they feel either it's not appropriate or necessary for them to express their identity, or they are fearful of surgical experiences, or there are health reasons. There are varied opinions as you will see from the following comments.

Heather. 'I hated my male body and that's the real reason why I chose to have reassignment surgery. I wanted to look in the mirror and feel comfortable with the silhouette that reflected the person I felt internally. But it's different for everybody. A person has to do what they feel is right for them because it's their life, their body and their pathway. What's right for one may not be the best choice for someone else. For me, I've had absolutely no regrets about having the surgery. I had talked my dysphoria through with my consultant and he appreciated that I hated my male-looking body. After discussing my personal history with him, he explained to me the choices available to me including the different types of operation and surgical techniques. He also fully explained the procedures available, risks and possible outcomes.

People often asked me how painful the surgery was. The truth is I only experienced moderate pain initially after the surgery and did not experience any complications afterwards. Most of my friends who also had full surgery would tell you the same and they had theirs done on the NHS. I went private, for two reasons. First, I could afford it and second I wanted to speed up the process and to start living my life properly. I had heard enough of the scare stories from the Gender Identity Clinic with my consultant informing me that hormone treatment would take ten years off my life span. My reply to him was that it would be ten less unhappy years. I took the same view with the surgery side of things and felt the need to proceed without taking too long to decide. I was nearly 40 at the time anyway. I know I'm lucky. There are many older trans women who can't have surgery because of medical problems – sometimes prevented by being overweight or heart or blood problems.

Having full reassignment surgery has made me far more expressive and outgoing than I was pre-transition years. It has simply boosted my confidence enormously.'

Tracy. 'I'm so glad I had surgery. I had my operation done in Thailand – but although I am pleased with the degree of my transition, I don't think that having surgery is the most important thing about transgender people. It's how you feel internally about yourself. Your self-confidence and belief in your gender identity is the most crucial element for your contentment and happiness.'

Odette. 'First of all, it is imperative to understand that any surgical procedure does nothing more than change an appearance. It does not change our gender, only our sexual identity. So, with it or without it, I am still female. That is my identity. But not having it does not make me less of a female.'

Lana. 'Surgery is a life-changing decision. It should never be taken lightly because there is no return once it is done, especially with genital reassignment before the person makes a final decision. The pros and cons must be fully explained to a person several times by a range of medical professionals.'

Molly. 'I remember being at a conference a few years ago and meeting a psychiatrist from the Leeds Clinic telling me that up to 25 per cent of his trans patients who had reassignment surgery regretted having it after three to five years. I was a little taken aback by this but I believed his sincerity. He went on to explain that for the first two years after a person has surgery they are in a state of euphoria because of the body changes, but gradually life does not turn out the way they had planned. The doctor said trans women in particular felt they were not accepted as women in society and also felt rejection from women who were cisgender. Others felt that their sexual relationships with men were not working out and others said they felt rejected by lesbians because of them being post-op. Patients went back to the doctor and told him they felt they had made a dreadful mistake having surgery and enquired about a reversal. But of course it is not possible – or at the very least it is immensely difficult to get a male body back once you have removed your penis and testicles. The only option open to trans people in this position is to accept it and to live life as best as possible.

I once told the story of what the psychiatrist told me on an internet forum but you should have seen the avalanche of abuse I received back telling me that I was ignorant, bigoted and so on and so forth. Personally I chose not to have reassignment surgery myself, partly because I felt I was too old for it by the time I transitioned in my fifties, but it is not something that I ever longed for anyway. I tire of hearing some trans women go on and on about having the op in order to complete their journey to the point they become fixated about the whole thing.'

One has to appreciate that this is Molly's viewpoint and experience, and that even if what the psychiatrist told her was true, the positive in this outweighs the negative in the sense that three out of four trans people are content with their surgery.

Trans women who came out in the 1970s know the difficulties, prejudices and obstacles better than anybody else. They have lived through tough times and paid a price for their bravery without compromising their desire to live authentic lives. The final two extracts in this chapter feature Georgina and Phoebe, just two of many women who have brought the rights of trans people into the public consciousness by merely being themselves and living open lives.

Georgina. 'It was the early '70s. I can still remember the flashing lights when the police came and arrested me. I was only taking a pee but somebody saw me and believed I was a flasher. They saw me as a man dressed as a woman. I guess I wasn't convincing enough in my new skirt and blouse. My secret was out and my parents threw me out, fully disowning me in the process. My friends became my new family but even they thought I was strange and difficult, but at least they didn't turn me away. There was no information about trans issues in those days, or at least it wasn't easily accessible. We have come a long way in 40 years, especially in legal terms. We no longer have to fight the law about which toilet we can use.

During my early years as transgender, I was constantly insulted and called a poof. I was often attacked but the police turned a blind eye because they didn't like people like me on the streets, so going out and staying safe was a struggle. I spent nearly 40 years living as a woman before I decided to have surgery. My only regret is that I didn't have it sooner.

Being in hospital made me realise that there are many trans people in the world, or at least that's how it felt when I met other men and women going through similar surgery. These days I am a happy and content person. I feel peace within myself. This is attributable to my feelings of being legal with my new birth certificate, passport and driving licence. In the last decade alone, I have witnessed a shift in the way society is becoming more tolerant and better informed about trans people through TV documentaries and the internet. I love going to Pride every year. Being seen in full public glare alongside many other trans people allows me to feel truly accepted, which in turn dispels the need to justify my existence.'

Phoebe. 'I began cross-dressing when I was aged six or seven while at primary school and even then I was very conscious that it was socially inappropriate. I felt suppressed having to remain closeted about my dressing. One day, when I was about 11, my brother walked in and caught me in my mother's dress and went straight and told our parents. "I'll stop this, I'll stop…", I promised them, trying to quench my embarrassment but I knew in my heart that this was the last thing I wanted to do. I continued with my dressing because this was the only way that I felt I could express my identity. It felt safe. It felt me. That horrible thought of being different temporarily ceased every time.

My father was a Methodist minister. I was raised with strong Christian views that I still hold to this day. We travelled around a lot which meant it became school after school, coupled with different homes, different neighbourhoods and different friends or, by the time of the seventh move, a complete lack of them. I was lonely. A friend would have been nice.

I recall the newspaper headlines and being on a tube in London when Renee Richards, the tennis player, underwent reassignment surgery in 1975. The whispers as passengers exclaimed at her photo, "Is that a man?" Her situation resonated with me more than anything else ever had. I was only 12 and filled with admiration for Renee, but I never thought I could equal her bravery.

Maybe, somewhere deep within my psyche, I knew that changing gender would never be easy. I was attracted to men through my adolescent years and when at university had many girlfriends. I still dressed up as often as I could but I was careful. I lived life most days as if nothing was wrong. The calmness of feeling all right in women's clothing was something I put to the back of my mind every time I changed back into men's clothes. In hindsight, perhaps I imposed this on myself. Maybe I was in denial. They were two different worlds. There was the one I inhabited and the other that I occasionally visited. It is difficult to articulate it now since I no longer live my life in this shadow.

I found in my earlier life I had to choose between my career and being different. I chose the former and went to university to study law. I now rationalise this mistake by differentiating the difference between knowing that you're different but not fully understanding the implications. I discovered, at great personal cost, that all the while I suppressed my true sense of self. I got married but I still cross-dressed. My wife accepted this to a point but insisted that I told nobody outside of our circle. In the days before the internet age, I bought alternative contact magazines, which helped me understand that there was a big bold world out there where others did what I did, and that I was far from being alone with my dark, murky secret. I started buying my own female clothing. This was the beginning of my new life and the beginning of the end of my marriage and former life as a man.

"This is not acceptable", was what my wife said when I told her that I wanted to become a woman. "Get out", were welcome words, in fact. It helped me in my journey towards becoming someone else. I was able to look in the mirror and for the very first time in my life say, with conviction, This is me.'

Finally, let me introduce you to Sophie who kept a diary on her journey to becoming a woman. She planned, she dreamed, and longed for the day to come when finally she would be able to go outdoors and be able to present herself to the world as a woman. Sophie prayed to be accepted. Here are some extracts from her diary:

- I came out to myself. Before that I was too frightened to talk to anyone about how I felt.

- I made the decision to become a full-time woman and I started dressing as a woman at home – but not at work as yet.

- I changed my name by deed poll, resulting in Steve becoming Sophie.

- I told my employer that I am a trans woman. They asked me many questions, for example, if I fancied any of the men at work and what toilet I wanted to use. I opted to use the disabled toilet.

- I went to my GP and told him I wanted to become a woman. He looked confused.

- After a third visit, my GP referred me to a psychiatrist. In fact I saw three in total before they deemed me mentally sane.

- I was referred to the Gender Identity Clinic.

- I attended the Gender Identity Clinic where I met many experts. I was asked many personal questions like, 'Were you interfered with as a kid?' and 'Are you a liar?' They made me cry. I was placed on hormone tablets which were gradually increased as time went by, but initially consisted of three months of injections and daily tablets.

- I received my Gender Recognition Certification and was then able to get a new birth certificate with my new gender stated on it.

- My burning aim is to have reassignment surgery. I know from the depths of my being that it will truly be the icing on the cake. For me, I will then be a complete woman.

Sophie isn't unique in making lists. In fact many trans people make lists, even if they are only a mental compilation of the things they need to do during the early stages of their transition. It marks the beginning of their new journey into the unknown. It's something they have thought about many times before finally finding the courage to become who they really believe they are; overcoming the many hurdles and obstacles that hinder their journeys but which, ultimately, pave the way towards them living the true authentic lives they feel are both their destiny and their entitlement.

CHAPTER FOUR

FEMALE TO MALE (FTM)

Aaron. 'I love cooking. My favourite type of music is Jewish rap. My clothes consist of tracksuit pants, trainers and tee shirts that are baggy and comfortable to wear. They help hide my breasts. I like Jean Paul Gaultier aftershave and my favourite film is *Man on Fire* starring Denzel Washington.'

Within the trans community, in the UK and Ireland, it is estimated that there are currently at least twice the number of trans women than there are trans men. However, more and more trans men are now coming out so the ratio is likely to become more balanced in future years.

History is sprinkled with stories of trans men serving in the army and navy in the 18th and 19th centuries. James Barry, from Ireland, who died in 1865, was a classic example. He was assigned female at birth but lived as a man for his whole adult life and became a renowned military surgeon in the British Army. Since gender reassignment hormones and surgeries were not available in that era, his lack of facial hair and high voice occasionally led to some people mocking his masculinity. However, he was nevertheless accepted as a man and it was only upon his death that he was found to have a female body.

Within the trans community trans men are often thought to have an easier time being accepted than trans women. This is largely because their appearance is not scrutinised as harshly and also because taking testosterone results in very effective masculinisation. However, while trans men may find it easier to blend in socially while clothed, those who want to modify the appearance of their genitals face more complex and risky surgery than trans women.

Trans men are currently more likely than trans women to begin their transitions at an early age and less likely to have previously married or to have had children.

Vinnie. 'I came out when I was aged 17, which is young, I guess. When I was ten, I knew that I was a boy. It felt so right, so proper for me to be so. But talking about puberty frightened me. I loathed such discussions but reconciled in my mind that I would get through it because I was a boy and that somehow I would bypass having periods and growing breasts because I would wake up one morning and I'd be a boy, having escaped the torture – although I hadn't worked out in my head how I'd achieve this.'

Although trans men are often assumed to simply seek to blend into society after transition these days, some are increasingly willing to identify publicly as trans and feel proud of who they are.

The relative lack of visibility of trans men compared to trans women within trans community spaces can sometimes leave trans men feeling isolated and misunderstood. Gradually trans men are building community spaces more specific to their needs while still recognising that trans people of all types need to work collaboratively in order to achieve full equality in society.

Owen. 'Trans women can sometimes, unintentionally, be unfair to trans men. I have often noticed support forums on the web where trans men post questions about transitioning out to the wider trans community. Comments like, "You are perfect as you are", aren't helpful. For some trans women, it's as if the penny hasn't dropped. They have the idea in their head to be female and somehow they fail to grasp that some women are actually men. Therefore, that's one of the main reasons why trans men often prefer to join support groups exclusively for themselves. Here they are free to discuss openly with other men the effects of taking testosterone whilst their periods continue, or problems with chest swelling following top surgery or even pregnancy, the storage of eggs prior to transitioning and trans-friendly midwives.'

The following extracts show how wonderfully accepting some families can be when a loved one comes out as trans – whilst the opposite applies in other cases. In Joshua's story, he was clearly accepted and loved by his parents and siblings. Darius and Ross were less fortunate and had to contend with rejection and prejudices from their mothers, but carried on regardless. This wasn't through stubbornness or some form of petty spite. Once they had begun their journey towards malehood, there was simply no turning back. They felt their maleness deeply and thwarted attempts to change them from anything that fell short of being a man.

Joshua. 'I had no language to express it. I was a boy with a female body who was attracted to girls. I hung out with the boys at school. They were cool with me and we often shared jokes about girls and who was hot – or not. The girls in my school took a different stance and were downright mean and nasty to me. They hated me sharing changing rooms with them because they thought I was looking at them when they were getting undressed. I often ended up changing in the toilets instead. But I knew I wasn't a lesbian because to be one, I would have to be a girl myself, which I knew I wasn't. Eventually, my parents allowed me to change to a private school that had no mandatory uniform. Here I was able to wear what I liked, usually a man's jumper and shirt.

When I was 16 I began reading up on trans issues. My laptop became an indispensable friend. I watched trans videos, trawled websites and devoured every word written about hormone treatments, surgeries and doctors. I decided to tell my GP. She was warm and kind towards me but admitted that she knew nothing about the subject. She asked me to return a month afterwards and that she would try her best to help me. I remember in the car on the way home my mother asking me, "What did you go to see the doctor about?" I told her I didn't want to say. "Was it to talk about having a sex change?" she asked. "Maybe…yeah", I replied. My mother replied, "Jesus Christ, I am your mother, you can tell me anything!" Then she told me how a week earlier she saw me walking towards the car through her wing mirror. It occurred to her how much I walked and looked like a boy – not a lesbian, a boy. I still remember her words, "It was a man walking towards the car."

Christmas Day came that year and after we had eaten our dinner, Mum announced to the family, "Have you anything to tell them?" First of all, I didn't quite understand and said "No", before realising what she meant. "Oh yes, I want to be a boy." "Is that all?", replied my brother. My sister was great too and joked how she'd always wanted another brother. I only ever felt love from my mother. She never said she felt like she was losing a daughter. I have gay friends who have told stories of coming out to their parents and being told that it felt like they were losing a child.

My advice to young trans men coming out is to be patient with the family and people you are coming out to. At first, they won't be able to understand things as you do because by the time you tell them, you have become an expert by everything you have Googled and read. I would also recommend that any person coming out should join a local support group for guidance, friendship and networking.'

Darius. 'People see trans men as masculine men and assume that they take hormones to look more masculine, whilst all along they are still lesbians. This is not true. They are men. Their brain is all male thinking, unlike lesbians who are not male and do not want to be male.

I grew up in rural Brazil and used to walk barefoot in the countryside without a shirt. Puberty started early for me with me getting my first period when I was nine. My mother told me to hide my chest. She encouraged me to play with my sister, who was very feminine, often comparing us and telling me to be more like my sister. I could not have imagined anything worse. I did not want to be like my sister in any shape or form. Instead, I made friends with other boys in the neighbourhood and together we played football and made kites.

When I arrived in Ireland, I decided to start my transition process. The first thing I did was start experimenting with names. I wanted to get used to people treating me like a man so I started using my new name on my Facebook page. Some friends sent me private messages telling me that I needed to seek out treatment and that I could be cured. But I knew there was nothing wrong with me and continued exploring hormone treatment and surgery.

I constantly try to educate others about trans people. Within the first half an hour of me meeting somebody new, I introduce the subject into our conversation. In doing so, I refer to my hormone treatment and this usually starts a conversation. I don't mind answering questions because there is little or no knowledge, not least any positive information that people know about trans people, so therefore it is only natural that they have much to enquire about.

My mother came over to visit me resulting in a showdown between us when one day she said to me, "You don't have to be a man to like girls." She said this over and over again despite my protests that I was not a lesbian, I was a man. She persistently called me by my old name. At one stage I was almost pleading with her to accept that I was her son but she did not relent. This got so heated that I warned her that unless she called me by my proper name or used the correct pronoun when referring to me, that I would ignore and not answer her when she spoke to me. Eventually this worked. These days she respects me more. At least this is how it appears outwardly but I know from looking in her eyes that me being a man still disturbs her a lot.

Dysphoria works differently for everyone – how you feel, how you like your body. Some people opt to have chest surgery, others genital reassignment. Here in Ireland, options for chest surgery are limited. There is a three year waiting list with the HSE (Ireland's public health service) and then the surgery you receive matches that of a cancer patient having a mastectomy. There is only one female surgeon in the country that carries out this procedure. Her specialism is with cancer patients and not trans men, hence this is a big problem with scar tissue and nipple reconstruction.

The vast majority of Irish trans men travel to Florida, where there are a range of specialist surgeons who are specifically trained to operate on trans men, or to some European country like Belgium or Germany. However, I am planning to go to Poland for my chest surgery. I befriended a trans guy on Facebook who was post-surgery. The first time I saw a picture of his chest, I said to myself, "Wow, he must have had this done in America." There was no visible scarring and his nipples were perfectly reconstructed. His chest was enhanced by hair which I thought looked incredibly sexy. He gave me the details of his surgeon, who I looked up on the internet. Now, I am saving up to travel to Poland. I am preparing for my surgery and have stopped smoking. Before I used to smoke a lot and the uncomfortable binding on my chest turned my posture into poor shape, so I started going to the gym and doing some exercise.'

Ross. 'The hardest bit at first was saying it out loud. When I was 11 I told teachers at school that I was a boy. The head teacher wrote to my parents expressing concern at what she considered unacceptable behaviour. In my twenties, I was in a straight relationship. My boyfriend wanted children, I didn't. It came to the point where I discovered that no matter how hard I tried to suppress my feelings, I always returned to questioning my identity. In the end, I came out to my boyfriend and although we split up, he was very supportive. We are still good friends. All of my other friends were great and full of encouragement towards my decision to transition.

My mother is an evangelical Christian. She deplored my transitioning and has never accepted it. To this day, she still calls me by my old name. I have got over it upsetting me and have come to terms with her disapproval. It wasn't such a big deal for my elderly father who told me that he had met people like me before. He offered me advice to be strong. Overall, my friends were amazing.

People feel trans people are a complete drain on the NHS. Certain sections of society are of the view that we cost billions because of hormone treatments, surgery and through Gender Clinics and psychiatrists. It is such a misleading conception because being trans is not a lifestyle choice. It is the opposite really in the sense that transitioning and all that it entails is necessary to free people from the unbearable mental torture that blights people for many years before they come to their decision to transition.

Transitioning to male has made me who I am today. It has made me the person I ought to have been all my life. I feel good with myself now like I never felt before. I now realise that my old life was never going to work. I was never a woman. Okay, I had the body of a woman but that is all. My mind – the way I thought – and the person inside were all male.'

Surgery

Like some trans women, there are some trans men who feel that surgery is not needed to relieve their dysphoria because gender distress is individual to every trans man. Some trans men have different priorities whereby some want their body characteristics to be congruent with how they identify. Some may be content with respect and pronouns. Most seek testosterone hormone therapy in order to significantly masculinise their face shape, hairline, body fat distribution and voice. Having breasts is often experienced as a particularly problematic incongruence because they are harder to ignore than the absence of a penis. Binding them in order to appear flat-chested can be painful and movement restricting. Therefore, chest reconstruction surgery is the most common surgery desired by trans men because the dislike of having breasts is arguably one of the biggest forms of dysphoria that trans men hold about their bodies.

Trans men with small breasts, 32B or under, can have liposuction to remove the breast tissue, which if successful leaves an excellent result and a masculine chest without any scarring. However, using liposuction to remove breast tissue is difficult, and some mammary gland tissues can remain, leaving the trans man retaining a later risk of breast cancer. For trans men the most common chest surgery is a bilateral mastectomy, which, dependent upon the size of the breasts, might also include removing, retaining and repositioning the nipples. The results can vary and, dependent upon breast size, most trans men will have some scarring, though it can line up with the under breast pectoral muscle line, making it a very successful aesthetic result. The benefit of a bilateral mastectomy is that it removes all of the breast mammary gland tissues, greatly reducing any future risk of breast cancer, though all trans men need to continue regular breast examination throughout their life.

Adam. 'It is easier to compensate for an absence but harder to suppress a presence. Every trans man does a spot of body mapping. I hated having breasts. They didn't fit with my sense of self. I viewed them as an unnecessary growth, and longed to return to the days of pre-puberty when I was flat-chested. Therefore, it was not a hard decision to have the lumps of fat removed. What was more difficult though was deciding whether I should take testosterone. I questioned if putting this chemical into my body was necessary for me to transition but knew there was no other means if I wanted to make my body look as masculine as possible. But as someone once remarked to me, "It is necessary to put petrol into a petrol engine – not diesel." The conflict was worth it because I am now very satisfied with how I look.'

Hysterectomy (the removal of the uterus and cervix) and oophorectomy (the removal of the ovaries) are usually recommended within the first five years of commencing hormone therapy, as there is some risk of developing pre-cancerous conditions of the cervix or ovaries. New laparoscopic techniques have made this much easier and far less physically traumatic than it was in the past, so even those trans men who are really into sporting activities or keeping fit can now undergo a hysterectomy and oophorectomy without fear of it affecting their fitness regime. Hysterectomy may be undergone together with the creation of a penis or as a stand-alone surgery. The main benefit of hysterectomy is that cervical smear tests will no longer be needed.

There are a variety of procedures which can be used to surgically create a micro-phallus or phallus (artificial penis) and simulated scrotum. However, phalloplasty and scrotoplasty currently require multiple surgeries and have significant frustrating limitations or risks associated with them. Trans men face having to decide what level of health risks they are willing to take. They also need to decide which factors are most important to them in regards to results: aesthetics, size, standing to urinate, sensation, erection ability, visibility of scarring and number of operations. It was often said that of the three key features trans men desire of a new phallus (looking good, urinating whilst standing up, and an erection for intercourse), they had had to choose two out of three, as creating all three within a new phallus was not possible. But recent advances in surgical techniques have meant that, within the last five years or so, a trans man can have an aesthetic phallus which enables him to urinate whilst standing and an internal erectile prosthetic that can be pumped up.

There is also the question of whether to have a vaginectomy (a surgical procedure to remove all or part of the vagina) or have the vagina occluded (closed up). For most trans men, this is a complex and difficult issue. Almost all trans men will say that they do not like having a vagina; some will actively hate the organ so much that they are desperate to have it removed. Other trans men will enjoy having their vagina penetrated during sexual activity. Others, even if not enjoying penetration, will recognise that, for them, the centre of their orgasm is contained within the vagina rather than the clitoris. It can be a very difficult decision to decide to lose those orgasmic abilities, especially as testosterone therapy increases the libido, so sexual activity, even if just masturbation, can be a very important part of the masculine identity of the trans man. The surgery is also complex and can lead to unsatisfactory consequences, so a considerable proportion of trans men who have had genital surgery will retain their former genitals, including their vagina and clitoris, behind their new phallus.

Even among those trans men who decide they want genital surgery, some still wait a number of years after transition before going for it in order to maximise their chance of benefiting from improvements in surgical techniques, and to ensure they have in place the support system they need before commencing such surgery. The many operations involved, and the very few surgical centres that exist, require trans men to be able to travel long distances post-operatively, which requires support and car transport wherever possible. Hospitals nowadays discharge patients, especially those who have had surgery, as quickly as possible, primarily to avoid patients becoming infected with MRSA or C. difficile. Consequently, recovery is mostly undertaken at home. The long and painful recovery times of the different phalloplasty stages require trans men to have a family or partner who can care for them whilst they are recuperating. And, very importantly, they need to have an employer who is understanding, and willing to allow them to take extensive and repeated periods off work during the surgery. The UK's Equality Act 2010 requires employers to allow time off and to pay trans employees who are undergoing gender reassignment treatment or surgery, at least during what would be the normal time periods for such surgery and recovery.

Despite all the advances in recent years in surgical techniques to create a phallus, almost all trans men who have undergone the surgery will have found some disadvantages, whether dealing with the problems of surgical failure, post-operative infection, long-term pain or sensitivity, or simply just very long recovery periods. A significant minority of these trans men will have had inter- and post-surgical complications, which in a few cases can result in lifelong disability. Consequently, some trans men decide against genital surgery, at least for the moment, instead being imaginative with their partner, making adjustments to their emotional understanding of their genitals or maybe using prosthetics instead of undergoing genital surgery.

Bruce. 'A man can be a man without a penis. For me, having a penis is not the defining feature of being male. A man is someone who is considerate, responsible. He is someone who looks out for others.

He is somebody who is chivalrous. He is accepted by society because he is looked up to by being a role model to others. I hope I am that man because I try hard to be.'

Freddie. 'I haven't ruled out ever having lower surgery, although I have read horrible stories, seen scary clips on the internet and know that having it done is extremely expensive. Politics and the NHS are far away from fully funding this type of surgery, which is incredibly invasive, on a frequent basis. I am looking forward to having top surgery, which I'm planning to have done in America in a clinic where they specialise in it. There will be quite a lot of scarring but, thankfully, my hormone treatment has enabled me to start growing hair on my chest so by the time of my surgery the scars that will run to under each of my armpits will be fairly well concealed by my chest hair.'

The following extracts expand further on the bravery of men who have transitioned and despite the challenges they have faced and continue to face, have found peace and acceptance within themselves. Rejection by family members is evident in Rory's life but the opposite is seen in Warren's story. A sense of loneliness is subtle but present in Blake, although his own sense of self-love continues to grow. Overall, these extracts, like the earlier three, show the determination and resilience exercised by these men who sought to live authentic lives in the gender they felt deprived of since birth.

Rory. 'I knew instinctively that there was something
different from an early age because I always took on
a male persona when I played games with my friends.
I was completely happy doing this. It felt completely
natural and, because of this relaxed attitude, my
friends were not bothered about it or indeed ever
questioned me. So in that sense there was no turmoil
because it wasn't a problem and therefore it wasn't
necessary to confide in anyone because there was no
secret to reveal.

When I reached puberty, reality took hold when
my periods started. What was happening to my body
felt so unnatural. I was horrified and disassociated
with every part of my body from my neck down.
The only slight relief was that I began to become
interested in boys. The fact that I was a gay male
teenager never occurred to me at that point because
my female friends too fancied boys, so nothing felt
unusual.

By the time I reached my early twenties, despite
feeling I was male, I attempted to suppress my feelings
and conform to how society usually expects young
females to behave. So I wore dresses and bought
make-up but loathed every aspect of the person I was
trying to emulate. It simply meant enduring a severe
level of frustration on a daily basis. I was wearing
a mask that was unbearable because there were two
dynamics constantly in battle with each other. One
part of me was desperate to pretend I was a woman
and the other part of me was equally as desperate to
come out and live my life as the man I was inside. But
my life was crumbling down because of my desperate
unhappiness. At some point, I began to realise that I

was never going to be happy unless I explored my gender in closer detail. But how? The answer in the end came relatively easily.

When I was in my early twenties, I went to Pride in San Francisco. This blew my mind away as I had never seen anything like this before in my life. It was colourful. It was fun. It was open. Here were people freely expressing who they were, without shame or inhibition, but more amazing were the crowds of people who cheered them on as they marched through the streets in their thousands. That liberated feeling will stay with me for ever. That was also the first time that I began to feel it was okay to acknowledge that I was trans. The first thoughts of it being all right for me to consider myself a gay man occurred too at this time. This simply became a time for me to explore my identity. I began spending more of my time in the gay community. I made friends easily through shared interests and similar outlooks on life.

After I returned home to Europe, I began my transition process. I joined a trans support group where I met other trans people. I was so quiet at first but it wasn't long before I started living my life the way I had wanted to live for many years. I gradually chose Rory as my name. It felt right. I was comfortable hearing people address me by it. Inner liberation continued and in a matter of weeks my confidence had grown. This newfound self-esteem and contentment coincided with a weekend trip away with the support group, where I met trans people from other groups and localities. Being in a group of like-minded people felt so right, so comforting, and made me realise that what I was doing was the right thing.

I bought a binder to hide my breasts. The first time I put it on, I remember looking in the mirror and liking what I saw. I smiled. I also bought a packer, a silicon penis and testicles which I slipped into my underpants. I had less success with this because there was a clip on it that constantly rubbed against my vagina. I cut my hair short and stopped wearing make-up. A new wardrobe loomed. So too did a trip to the charity shop with my old clothes.

I went to my GP and told him about my transition process. I began to look into the medical side of it. My doctor advised me to see a psychiatrist to ensure that what I was doing was the right thing. Sensibly, the psychiatrist recommended counselling and for this I am grateful. After I started taking hormones, my emotions were all over the place. At the same time, I was dealing with family issues – ridicule and rejection about what I was doing. Coping with this hostility and the effects of the hormones on my body, I found counselling was a great way to share my thoughts and helped to make sense of them. It is certainly something I suggest to other trans people who begin hormone therapy. I consider counselling essential to guide you through the process because no matter how much you think before transitioning that you are doing the correct thing, once the hormones take effect, there will be moments of confusion and doubt.

My friends accepted the new me but the same didn't apply to my family. My mother was horrified when I started transitioning. It became a daily ritual for her to say, "What will people think or say? Whatever will they think of me as a parent?"

But mostly she coped by refusing to talk about it or acknowledge that I had become a man. I developed acne in the early stages of taking hormones. One day I mentioned a big spot I had on the side of my nose. My mother asked what could have caused it. I said it was probably a side-effect of the hormones. She pursed her lips. Silence fell on the room before she changed the conversation.'

Warren. 'Will I pass? Won't I pass? Will society accept me or not? These are never-ending questions. Being trans is part of my history. It is also part of my present. I am different to someone who was born male. Because for 20 years of my life I was socialised in a different way to cisgender men, therefore I have a different perspective of the world. In many ways, life is about closing the gap between being a man and being a trans man. I am fortunate to pass easily as a man, and have never hidden from people the fact that I was born a woman. Although I want people to first and foremost see me as a man; I want them to recognise the experiences I have as a trans man. However, setting out to mark this difference does not mean that I am ever inviting them to see me as a female, because I'm not. The end point here is that I am male but I was not born male and therefore I request that society recognises this difference. This means, for my part, that I must be upfront about my experiences.

I didn't have a conventional childhood. Of course, I disliked girl's clothing, toys and playing silly girly games. It never felt right, but I did not know what was different about me. You will find some trans men who will tell you that they knew by the age of three that they were not female, but I personally think that it is something individual to each person and many others will be older or well into their teens before they have cognition as to who it is they are. It is different for everyone because it takes each individual to make sense of it by themselves. Nobody else can do this for you because it is only you who knows you and who can make sense of you.

I remember going into the toilets one day when I was at university. There was only one other man in there. He suddenly turned towards me and challenged me on my gender. I told him I was male but he refused to believe me. "Pull down your trousers", he demanded. I refused and after a further exchange of words, I made a hasty retreat. In hindsight, anything could have happened to me. He might have beaten me, tried to rape me or, if I hadn't left, he might even have attempted to pull down my trousers. It was a horrible experience and brought home to me the hazards that some trans men face in society.

My mother is the most amazing woman I have ever met and the most loving. When I was 22, she said to me, "Have you ever thought about becoming a boy?" Although I had from time-to-time considered transitioning, there was something pivotal in her words that made me think more seriously about that matter, especially as her reassurance that she and my father would be absolutely fine about it should I decide to do so. I went to a counsellor to discuss it further. It wasn't long afterwards that I realised that Mum was correct and thereafter I set upon a pathway that I have never regretted.'

Blake. 'My life prior to transitioning was horrible. I was depressed and suicidal and spent time in a psychiatric hospital. I have a mild learning difficulty and didn't cope well at school. I had family issues and argued with them all the time. I hated myself. I hated my body. I didn't have many friends. Then I watched a documentary called *My Transsexual Summer* on Channel Four and around the same time there was a storyline in *Hollyoaks* about a trans person. These helped me recognise myself better. Although I always knew I was male, a little voice at the back of my head used to tell me that I could change my identity from a woman into a man. Coming out was painful and caused even greater friction and distance between me and my family but once I started transitioning, I never wanted to turn back. Testosterone saved my life really, in the sense that it helped me start the journey to release the real me. I am having top surgery in the coming months to remove my breasts.

I am a gay man and although I have not yet had the confidence to pursue a relationship, this is not something I have ruled out but I would like to wait until my top surgery is complete and healed. From an early age, I have always been attracted to males, but never from a female point of view. I get on with men as a man in a way that I could never relate to them as a woman, mainly because I used to never wear female clothes prior to transitioning. In this sense, my wardrobe has hardly changed because I have always worn trackies, hoodies, jeans and trainers.

I have always been good at sport, particularly athletics and football. I like to keep fit and in good shape. I'm not saying that I have a six-pack yet but, who knows, maybe I will have one day. The discomfort of binding my breasts will then be gone. I will no longer have to look at them with resentment. It will make sports easier too, although all my teammates know that I am a trans man and fully respect me. My team and I represented Great Britain in athletics in the last Special Olympics and we won silver.

I have my own flat now and am beginning to look forward to the future. These days I have made lots of new friends through college and in the trans support group and LGBT group that I've joined. We socialise and have great fun amongst ourselves. In my dreams, I have forgotten the female version of me. She hardly existed, though. I see myself totally as a man despite my female body parts. If there was better education in society about trans people, then barriers would get broken down and coming out may not be so hard.'

To conclude this chapter, I will focus on older trans men. As mentioned earlier, many from previous decades transitioned to malehood and then afterwards lived their lives in total privacy. They knew from an early age that they were never supposed to be women and chose to distance themselves from this gender role as best they could whilst superficially remaining within the confines of society at the time. Coming *out* was often very difficult for them, but many would say that not having legal equality or recognition meant their lives were even more difficult before they came out and started the battle for better legislation and recognition of the human rights of trans people. In recent years there has also been an increase in the number of older trans identified wo/men, who have often had children, finally deciding to seek gender reassignment treatment and transitioning to live in their new gender role. Many other older trans men have since returned to the trans community and are sharing their experiences and wisdom with younger trans men. One of these men is Liam and here are some of his reflections on his life.

Liam. 'When I was born, my mother described her life as a coma of happiness. After having six boys, I was now her little girl and was someone she had longed for all her life. But I was never destined to be a girl. I hated girls' dresses. I had absolutely no interest in my hair, preferring it short and straight. Whenever I was given a doll as a present, I threw it away in a fit of temper. I think even as a young child I would have passed as a boy. I was always friends with boys in my local area, which my brothers hated and often cruelly tried to bully me into playing with girls instead.

At home, I constantly battled how I felt and how others perceived me, but by the time I was eleven I had worked out what was really going on inside me. This was greatly helped by a magazine my mother bought that contained an article about a man who went and had a sex change in London. It hit a raw note but also it helped me piece my identity together. I remember cutting out the article and hiding it under my bed, often returning to read it over and over again.

When I was 12, a teacher remarked to me, "You look like a boy, you don't look like a girl." I looked at her in silence. I have always loved traditional male interests – bikes, planes, football, cowboys and reading about wars. Indeed, it was my love of books that I often used as a camouflage to my identity. People just assumed that I was clever and odd, yet accepted this as part of somebody who liked reading and was clever. By the time I was 13, I had horrible thoughts of one day having to get married to escape detection. As I grew older I started to plan my escape to London where I intended to have a sex change operation. Life ticked by in the meantime with much isolation and secrecy. I had few friends at the time so I knew my change of gender would not affect them, but there were moments I wondered how my family would react, how I would tell my mother and if I would lose them all as a result. But these intense inner feelings were coupled with thoughts of how liberated and free I would be after surgery.

The only drawback to my plan was my lack of money so I formed another plan. I decided that when I went to England, I would study electronics at college so that I could become a radio officer in the Merchant Navy. The folly of youth filled my mind with nonsense. For some reason I thought I'd be able to travel on a different ship for each voyage. Something told me that you got long holidays in the navy so I figured out that this would be ideal, giving me the opportunity to have surgery in-between trips before joining a different ship and crew where nobody would notice any difference in my appearance. None of this happened though because when I turned 20, I went to England and ended up working in a bank instead.

Every day I went to work and presented as a female but inwardly I felt male. I knew I had a body I did not want and eventually decided to go to my

GP and tell him that I wanted to become a man. I described to him how I felt trapped in the wrong body. He said he had heard of transsexuals but had never met one before. He referred me to a psychiatrist who in turn referred me to Dr John Ransdell, who at the time was the leading trans specialist at the Charing Cross Clinic. He was a fearsome man, blunt and rude, who tried and tested my willpower in every aspect to see if I would break under his challenging of my gender. He basically wanted to see if I really was a man or whether it was some grand illusion I had about myself. When he deemed me sane, our relationship improved. He told me that I needed to pass as a man and in order to prove myself that I needed to undertake a manual job for a year.

I got a job on a building site which from the very outset was a farce. I hated practical work, much preferring academia, but I tried to be as macho as possible. Whilst nobody detected my birth gender, my skills on the construction site were limited. When somebody passed a remark about this, I lamented with great pretence that my father died when I was a young boy and that was the reason why I was never taught practical, manual tasks. Thankfully, I was believed and eventually got through the year, but little did the men at work know that I lived in Balham in a house along with other transsexuals.

My next awakening arrived shortly after I left the building site when I commenced hormone therapy and grew facial and body hair. This made me feel more masculine than my previous butch persona, with my life feeling more complete than it had ever been before.'

CHAPTER FIVE

NON-BINARY

Blair. 'My mind tells me that I am neither female nor male. If you read me as a woman, that's fine, but please don't tell me that I am a woman. Call me a man…well, that feels wrong somehow because I don't look like a man nor do I feel I'm a man. There have been lots of people who insist on telling me that I couldn't possibly be non-binary, but they are basing this entirely on how they perceive me. There are others who insist that I must be a lesbian, but I have never had a sexual relationship with a woman. I'm not ruling it out one day, but so far this has not been part of my story. It is difficult to be around people who don't know I am non-binary or with those that challenge its existence. I can only compare to how some gay people feel they are not themselves when they are around their parents who they haven't told, or with work colleagues who don't know, or with acquaintances who might assume that the gay person is straight and treat them as such.'

Aiming for neutrality

A large majority of cisgender people and indeed many people within the LGBT framework – including some trans men and trans women – will never have heard of non-binary people or understand what this entails. The key defining feature of a non-binary person is that they do not feel comfortable thinking of themselves as simply either a man or a woman. They reject the traditional Western idea of gender as binary, defined only in terms of man or woman. Instead they feel that their gender identity is more complicated to describe. It is important to remember that being a non-binary person is not the same thing as being an intersex person, because non-binary is about the way someone self-defines their gender identity while intersex is about the physical body a person is born with.

Some non-binary trans people may identify their gender as a mixture of being a man and a woman or as fluctuating between man and woman. Alternatively, they may feel they have no gender and prefer simply to be seen as just a human being. Admittedly, this can be confusing for the person and also for partners, family and general members of society to understand and appreciate.

Non-binary trans people span a wide range of desires to transition. Some have no interest in undergoing any form of gender reassignment. Others may wish to partially transition for example, a non-binary person assigned female at birth may undergo chest reconstruction but will still continue to reject identifying simply as a man or as a woman.

Drew. 'Thirty years ago, people wouldn't have the option of being non-binary because there was so much pressure to be binary. Some transitioned to opposite gender and although most found satisfaction, you may question that, if the option had been available, would some of those people have opted to be non-binary?'

Labels

Although most people who identify as non-binary trans people are young, there are some older people in this category as well. However, new vocabulary and terminology is being formed by younger people who communicate with other non-binary people through online blogs and discussion groups on Facebook. Other social media networks, like Tumblr, prove particularly popular amongst this group.

Sky. 'We young non-binary people are testing new language and creating our own words. I don't like the word "biological". Assigned at birth is more encompassing because that is what the person was given at the time – they had no choice in the matter. This was based on their physical traits. Nobody was prepared to keep an open mind. Whilst older people are generally rigid in the way they think about gender, I think children should be taught to have an open mind – male, female or other.

I became aware of my gender dysphoria when I was 16, although at school and all through growing up my best friends were boys. I loved football and masculine things. I remember sex education in school and thinking how unfair everything was in life. I didn't want puberty to happen. I resented the physical things that started to occur. I was more curved than I wanted to be but I didn't feel like a girl and neither did I feel like a boy and had no craving to become one. Although I associated mainly with boys growing up, these days I feel uncomfortable being alone with men because I feel there is a lack of acceptance, especially from older cisgender men who I have received most criticism from in the past.'

Overall the number of non-binary people is low but the following list shows the number of personal identities is continously growing, although the most common are gender-queer, gender-fluid, gender-variant and agender:

- Agender or non-gender – no gender expression and/or no gender identity.

- Androgyne – possessing simultaneously masculine and feminine traits.

- Bigender – someone who has two separate genders. Male and female are but one example of the two genders.

- Demiboy – someone who only partially (not wholly) identifies as a boy or man, whatever their assigned gender at birth. They may or may not identify as another gender in addition to feeling partially a boy or man.

- Demigirl – someone who only partially (not wholly) identifies as a girl or woman, whatever their assigned gender at birth. They may or may not identify as another gender in addition to feeling partially a girl or woman.

- Gender-fluid – a person who feels like a mix of traditional male and female genders but on some days feels more traditionally male gendered and others more traditionally female gendered.

- Gender-fuck – is the practice of bending stereotypical gender appearances and mannerisms, resulting in a mixture of masculinity and femininity (for example a person with a beard wearing a dress).

- Gender non-conforming – a broad term that covers all the individuals who appear and behave in ways that, according to society's expectations, are atypical for one's originally assigned gender role.

- Gender-questioning – a person who is currently questioning or experimenting with gender identity.

- Gender-variant (similar to gender non-conforming) – expression by an individual that does not match cultural expectations about the gender role that was assigned to them at birth.

- Gender-queer – the state of being beyond or between genders or a combination of genders. The term pushes back against the social construct aspect of the gender binary system, gender stereotypes and gender itself.

- Inter-gender – a person whose gender varies from the traditional norm, or who feels their gender identity is neither female nor male, both female and male or a different gender identity altogether.

- Neutrois – a term used to describe persons with a null or neutral gender (being neither male nor female), and in some cases, a person who may seek to reduce signs of their physical sex.

- Non-binary – not part of the male/female gender binary (a binary is limiting because it has room for only two categories, and those categories must be opposites.

- Pan-gender – people who reject the male/female gender binary because they feel that they are all genders.

- Trans-feminine – an inclusive term for a trans person who is currently feminine of centre in identity or presentation.

- Trans-masculine – an inclusive term for a trans person who is currently masculine of centre in identity or presentation.

Non-binary gender identities are not a new abstract concept, although society has always been binary focused. There will always have been people who have felt not entirely male, or not entirely female, or have felt they were both genders. The concept of being androgynous has come more prominent in the trans community in recent times with some people presenting as neither clearly masculine nor clearly feminine in appearance, which is the prime aim for a great many non-binary people. Society is now seeing far fewer people feeling trapped in binary gender categories. This has resulted in far less anxiety for the person experiencing this internal friction. Some non-binary people have even felt that by simply acknowledging their identity to themselves alone brought them great inner peace and was the beginning of their transition.

Outside of non-binary circles but within the broader trans community, there are those who find that too many labels cause confusion and uncertainty in the LGBT community, and also amongst the general population. Some may complain that the list of different identities within the non-binary framework is too large or even nonsensical.

Keegan. 'The issues around redefining gender labels could lead to greater discrimination for some individuals who don't conform to understandable gender expressions. These labels might be okay in colleges or universities, but in everyday workplaces they may find less tolerance and acceptance.'

A counter argument against having too many labels is that some consider it comforting to find a label that they feel best resembles who they are. Others say having a label that best describes them gives a clear and accurate meaning to the ways they themselves wish to identify and how they wish to identify to others.

The following extracts explain how labels have helped people understand themselves better in putting their gender identity into context.

Harper. 'I think the easiest description is that I don't feel I fit or belong in either the female or the male box. Neither label properly describes how I feel inside, like a shoe that just doesn't fit the shape of my foot. Before starting to identify as non-binary, I identified as trans man for a few months, but the cultural baggage and narrative that came with internally identifying with that label didn't feel significantly better than identifying as female. I see an explicit difference of feeling between internal and external identification, because I still present to the cisgender world as male, but now that I'm not internally identifying with it, I don't feel in myself that huge weight and normalising pressure that I felt when I did internally identify with maleness.'

Amaris. 'When I was due to hit puberty, I wanted to take oestrogen. I wanted to be a grown-up so that I could be independent. I do think I also wanted to be a proper woman and I wanted people to stop asking me what I was and making fun of me. I thought that if I looked more like a woman, they would stop. As it turns out, it didn't stop me being made fun of. I just got made fun of for supposedly being a lesbian. Not to mention, I've been struggling with my body since I grew breasts. I'm currently seeking a reduction. I didn't discover the term "gender-queer" until I was around 17. Now I identify more as non-binary because gender-queer seems to have a fluidity that doesn't reflect me. I don't feel like my gender is fluid or has changed from the beginning. I have always been how I have been. The only difference is that I have the words to describe it now.'

Description within labels

A description within a label has the added value of people having to ask fewer questions because much of the information is evident within and this prevents unwanted questions. Having said that, people outside the trans community will still ask questions but these labels and descriptions are infrequently used in the cisgender world.

Riley. 'Each and every one of us is unique. Realistically, everyone falls into each of these different categories, whether they realise it or not. It is unrealistic to label everyone within the binary constraints of male and female. Therefore, it is completely realistic that we have so many categories. What is unrealistic is having to choose between just two genders.'

Zuriel. 'I hear a lot of people say, "Why have labels, I'm just human?", and that aggravates the hell out of me. Labels help explain things. Or at least they give you something to relate to. And I like that. So it makes me feel good to have that. I am agender. I don't feel like I have any gender. I don't feel like I'm gender non-conforming. I look like a woman and I feel like the only way to be non-conforming is to be more masculine and I have no desire to be masculine.

I don't know if there's something in my brain that makes me different to binary identified trans people or cisgender people. I don't really care. I don't think we know enough about the brain to say for sure. And I don't think it matters either way. My identity is legitimate regardless of whether it is biological or not. The only battles I've had to fight have been the ones with people about them coming to terms with me being non-binary – or not. I don't specifically present as anything anywhere. I am who I am.

I wear what makes me comfortable and happy. People assume I'm a woman and at work I don't bother correcting them because I don't have the patience or time to explain myself to them. I don't feel like I need people at work to gender me correctly to feel happy with who I am.'

Sasha. 'We have to look at the scientific laws of the universe and when we do we'll start to realise that matters relating to identity won't become simpler as time goes by. Some might say that having to prove gender identity is part of oppressive structure within society, whilst others feel okay with labels because it helps them understand the identity of others. At the moment, we perhaps have too many labels and words in the non-binary community that appear alien to the cisgender world. I appreciate this must be confusing at times but the problem is that it is virtually impossible to settle on one simple narrative to explain trans issues. I know some trans people dislike us because they feel we don't take the issue of being trans seriously enough, and criticise us for not knowing who we are. Then there are cisgender people who argue with us and ridicule us for not being able to identify with either gender, and it angers them that we don't make a concerted effort (as if it is that easy) to identify with the gender in which we were assigned at birth.'

The following extracts from Brady, Robin and August provide greater clarity into their journeys of discovering who they really are and what description best applies to each one individually.

Brady. 'I've had these feelings all of my life. I told my mother when I was 16. She was not bothered and basically accepted me as I am. When I was 18, I dressed entirely in female clothing and was addicted to wearing make-up. I wouldn't look at myself in the mirror until I was wearing it. Being gender-fluid entails never sticking to a particular gender for long because two years later I grew a beard and started identifying as more masculine. I am naturally quite effeminate and people often confuse me as being merely gay.

With regard to sexuality, I identify as pansexual. Currently I am in a relationship with another non-binary person who identifies as trans-masculine. Although assigned female at birth, he too has experienced people assuming that he is a lesbian. That's the problem with making assumptions because by doing so, you miss out on discovering the real identity of the person.

I identify as a non-binary feminine person. Or just as non-binary. The feminine part of it is pretty important as that's how I present myself and move through my life. There are other words that affect my gender identity that I attach onto this descriptor (depending how I'm feeling on the day or what space I'm explaining my gender identity in).

I've always thought that there are as many gender identities as there are people. For people unfamiliar with each identity there might be no differences between them, but for people to whom those words mean something, there can be important differences. Many people try out a few terms and decide one or more fits them, other terms change meaning as conversations develop in a wider context. The language around trans identity within trans communities is an ever-shifting landscape and a minefield.'

Robin. 'I was assigned female at birth and I wasn't consciously aware of my gender dysphoria until the age of 23. I remember I always hated it when boys and girls were explicitly or subtly separated for activities either in school or in the family (e.g. at family gatherings – women and girls grouped in the kitchen, men and boys in the garden). And I always hated it when I felt people treated me differently because I was a girl/woman, but part of this was probably due to living in a sexist society.

I also always had an aversion to my breasts, but in the narrative I grew up with, there was no such thing as a woman who would hate her breasts, so I ignored my feelings about this, aside from my slight bafflement when my (cis) male partners seemed to like them. Also, I always envied boys' and men's physiques and the fact that they are stronger and faster than women without needing to put any effort into achieving it.

I use agender, or if I really want to go into detail, trans-masculine agender. I mean by it that I don't feel I have an internal gender, just a slight masculine tone. Also I use trans-masculine to state that I was assigned female and transitioning to a masculine role and body. I used to identify for about a year as gender-fluid, as my internal sense of gender was shifting among male, genderless (agender) and gender-queer, but for about 18 months now this shifting has stopped and left me without any internal feeling of gender, so nowadays I generally use agender.'

August. 'When I was a child I was very much a tomboy. I occasionally experimented with femininity, because that's what was expected of me; however I was always happiest being one of the boys. However, I was completely unaware that it was possible to be non-cisgender. I didn't even know the word "transgender". I always assumed I was just a more masculine girl.

When I reached puberty, about the time I started secondary school, I hated what was happening to my body. My mother has particularly vivid memories of me crying and being extremely confused, telling her that it was unfair and that I didn't want it to happen. But I figured everyone felt that way, other girls were just better at coping with it. I had regular feelings of what I now recognise as gender dysphoria, particularly strong feelings of discomfort with the shape of my body. I was just shy of 16 when I had my "Eureka, I'm trans!" moment.

I have found real peace, real harmony, since I accepted that the term "non-binary" best fits my identity. I've met so many great people, with such a wide range of interests, and there are so many people willing to help, willing to listen and understand because we have shared experiences and feelings. Particularly in the online community, there's a great sense of comradeship and unity. I've learned so much about politics, history and issues around the world, because of being non-binary.'

Acceptance and pronouns

As you have read there are many identities within the non-binary framework, although a large number of people do not go into detail about their individual preference and simply say they are non-binary. Having said that, a common expression of identity expressed by others is that of gender-queer.

Ollie. 'Gender-queer is my gender identity. As a gender-queer person, I don't see myself as either male or female, but rather a blur between the two. For me, personally, I like my female physicality and embrace my masculine mentality. My stereotypically male characteristics of thought and expression are important to me, but unlike a trans man, I have no desire to alter my body to match. I prefer gender neutral pronouns, they/their/them.'

As with Ollie, the use of pronouns is very important to non-binary people. Respecting non-binary gender identities is equally important to respecting all other aspects of people's identities. Therefore, it is important to use the name, title and pronouns that a non-binary person requests. The gender neutral pronoun *they* is most often requested by non-binary people. Other terms are *fey*, *per*, *xie* and *zie*. These terms are personal pronouns used as a substitute to standard pronouns like *he* or *she* and *him* or *her*.

Looking beyond addressing non-binary people in person, there comes the matter of how to address a non-binary person during correspondence, particularly in a formal nature. It may cause offence to address them as

Mr, Miss or *Ms*. It is considered best to leave out titles when addressing non-binary people unless they have already told you which title they want you to use. They are increasingly using gender neutral titles like *Misc* or *Mx*.

Curtis. 'It doesn't bother me any more but I would like a third gender marker on official documents. I would like to use the Mx neutral title because this is the one I use for other trans people that I know. Non-binary is a useful umbrella term. I actually prefer gender-queer myself, and my research tells me it's the majority preferred term for self-identification; but it's also felt to be offensive by some non-binary people and is less likely be taken seriously by cis people, so using non-binary is more politically correct within the trans community.

Terms are not very important to me. I don't often talk about my gender identity day-to-day – I don't imagine most cis people do either. It's useful to apply such categories for research and political purposes but day-to-day I'm just me and the people around me know what that means.'

Jordan. 'I feel sad for non-binary people who are still stuck on visibility and who feel like they need wider recognition via the State. While I think it would be nice to be able to have myself formally recognised for who I am in some capacity (e.g. removing my gender marker from my documents, choosing a gender neutral title), I don't think that I need that in order to be happy. Life is short. I really don't see a purpose in trying to convince a society of my worth and value, because when I look at this society there's so many different types of discrimination that exists. I don't think it's worth my time to appeal to society to recognise me.'

Identity

Imagine walking down a street where most of the time you will correctly assume the gender identity of those around you. Occasionally, somebody's gender will appear ambiguous. It is then that you might look closely for signs, for example, breasts or a bulge in the crotch area. But in these circumstances no matter how much you try to discern that person's gender, you may never know for certain unless you ask, which might be rude or intrusive. The person whose identity has confused you may not even be trans.

Admittedly, it often causes huge upset for cisgender people to be mis-gendered but this is sometimes an everyday occurrence to trans people. The main point here is that identity is unique and personal to each person, and to remember appearance is one thing and what a person's brain tells them they are is quite another.

Presley. 'Stop taking it as an insult. Be okay if people ask about your identity and what pronouns you prefer. It's not a big deal – or at least not for me. Anyway, I always know whether somebody asking a question is genuinely sincere in wanting to understand my trans identity or some other aspect of the trans community. If I sense insincerity, sarcasm or rudeness, I usually shut the conversation down pretty quickly.'

In most countries it is not possible for non-binary people to get gender neutral birth certificates or passports. Likewise, society is structured on the assumption that there are only men and women, so there is usually no provision for access to (non-disabled) gender neutral toilets and changing rooms or non-binary titles or *no title* forms and documents. They find it unfortunate to think that their core essence is misunderstood and is mainly unaccepted through ignorance.

Taylor. 'I dress androgynous – never overly masculine and never feminine. My hair is short. I love bright colours and presently my hair colour is pastel pink. These days you will find me dressed in jeans, checked shirt, hoody or a tee shirt with some kind of movie reference logo on it. Sometimes, I wear a bow tie, which is a popular choice with non-binary people, and a pair of doc martens. I never wear make-up.'

Nikki. 'There is more acceptance now than we would have received 20 years ago when society had a clear rule – pink for girls and blue for boys. They forgot a third colour for people like me. And although the world has stormed ahead with change, many feel that when it comes to gender, it has gone backwards.'

Ashley. 'I don't identify with men. Neither do I identify with masculinity – for example, the stereotypical notion of not being emotional in public, or not crying easily and not being able to tell someone the reason when you are upset. I dislike men who are loud, abrasive and those who use their strength for sexual violence.

I don't feel I belong amongst women either. I detest the way that it never occurs to cisgender women that there are other women in the world who are different to them. I worry the moment I am amongst women how they will perceive me because they never fail but to mis-gender me. I fear the questions they will ask and the assumptions they'll make. Neither do I enjoy being around lesbians. They rarely understand non-binary people who were assigned female at birth because mentality is rigid towards their own gender identity and sexuality.'

Bowie. 'I only faced a battle when I was trying to be female. I have absolutely no difficulty simply being myself. At the point of self-acknowledgement it forces one to rethink one's life and question one's prejudices about gender. I find it much easier to like women now I'm not trying to be one.'

This chapter closes by looking at an extract from Cassidy and the struggles *they* have endured to make sense of *their* binary identity. The overriding theme is of an ongoing journey of self-acceptance, with the aim of arriving at a point where Cassidy feels completely at ease with *their* identity.

Cassidy. 'Gender issues never really crossed my mind until I was 16 or 17. Before that I thought I was a gay man. It was not until a few of my friends came out as being trans and, around the same time, I started having a sexual relationship with a lesbian friend. Initially I thought I was bisexual or pansexual, but that did not ring true. The more I looked inwardly at myself for answers, the more I was drawn towards the idea that I was trans. After this clicked in my head the floodgates opened.

At first I started to transition to being a woman. It didn't feel right, though, as I did not feel like a woman and, furthermore, my inclinations to become a woman were not strong. But I didn't feel like I was a man either and my inclinations to wanting to be a man were equally weak. I questioned if I was in fact a gender-queer man and sought to live as one for a period. That didn't work. After considering a few other labels I settled on non-binary as the more I thought about my identity, the more I was drawn towards neutrality.

For me, the sensible aim is to look as androgynous as possible. I take a low dosage of hormone therapy that will eventually make me look neutral. I don't want breasts but neither do I want to look flat-chested. This is, in the main, the goal for most non-binary people, with the exception of those who consider themselves to be gender-fluid and bi-gendered.

Although gender identity doesn't have anything to do with genitals, I still have dysphoria about my genitalia. I hate my penis but have no desire to have a vagina either. But take a trans woman, for example, who does not opt to have lower surgery, that doesn't compromise her position as a woman. My dislike of myself stems from the fact that I was gendered as male at birth and subsequently socialised as male, and the more I think about this, the more I veer away from being male and the more I veer towards being a woman, and the more my brain tells me that I am not a woman and neither do I want to be one.

At the moment, I present as less male and that sometimes means that people assume I am female. I don't necessarily take umbrage at this and, although I don't identify with being female, I nevertheless do not have the same degree of emotional baggage with this as I do with being called a man. Shaving is hell that I could do without and wearing make-up is a boring but necessary chore to hide any remaining stubble. But it's all about getting to a comfortable level with how I think about myself and to become more comfortable with my body. That way, there is less emotional angst and although I don't always feel comfortable with myself, it does not grate against me in the same manner as my assigned gender at birth.

Unlike some trans women and men, who decide to live their lives in a stealth manner, I have to be open to people about my identity because otherwise they will incorrectly gender me, which causes embarrassment and sometimes upset, especially around toilet usage. Unlike trans women and men, non-binary people do not have gender identity certificates, so using female toilets is my preferred choice if the establishment I'm visiting does not have disabled facilities.'

CHAPTER SIX

CROSS-DRESSERS

First of all let me clear up any confusion that might surround drag artists, trans women and cross-dressers. Drag artists and trans women are the best known groupings from the main trans categories. Nearly everyone will have seen a man in drag, either on television, in a nightclub or in panto. They are mainly men dressed as women; occasionally women dress as men – drag kings. The intention of drag artists is to be theatrical – camp and comical, with exaggerated feminine expressions. It is intended as a harmless performance for the purpose of entertainment. It does not reveal the performer's personal gender identity or how they live their day-to-day life. This is in contrast to a trans woman who does not dress as a character nor perform a gender role for entertainment; she dresses as herself and simply seeks to live her daily life as the person she presents as all the time. Cross-dressers are neither drag artists nor trans women (the number of female cross-dressers is minute in comparison to males).

A cross-dresser is someone who wears clothing traditionally associated with a different gender but usually does not wish to transition permanently. They may cross-dress in order to express a different side of their personality, to escape temporarily from their day-to-day life stresses, or simply to feel more comfortable or confident. In such cases, their cross-dressing may be quite frequent and public. For others, cross-dressing may be a very private action as part of erotic role-play or sexual arousal. For some, however, cross-dressing is a prelude to transition, as their discomfort with the gender role assigned at birth becomes more intense.

The extent, frequency and visibility of being a cross-dresser differs widely for each person. Some men wear only one item, for example, female knickers or hosiery under their male clothes. Other men dress head to toe in female clothing, including make-up and wigs. They adopt a female persona which they refer to as their alter-ego which involves giving themselves a female name. There are cross-dressers who dress in the privacy of their own homes or in a hotel room. Others are more narcissistic in nature. They love to be seen dressed in their female clothing in public and some like having their pictures taken.

When people hear about transvestites and cross-dressers they sometimes wonder about the difference between the two. Some trans people believe there is not any dissimilarity between both. Others say transvestites are individuals who wear clothing of the opposite gender for erotic arousal or sexual gratification, although some do so for emotional or psychological reasons as well, especially as they get older. Cross-dressers on the other hand are believed to dress in female clothing in order to satisfy an intense feminine side of themselves, in a way they feel they would otherwise not be able to do. Sexual gratification does not appear to be part of this, although many say that they started by stealing their mother's or sister's underwear and masturbating while wearing them, but later grew out of any sexual arousal from cross-dressing.

Some trans people consider the term 'transvestite' to be old fashioned. These days the term 'cross-dresser', which was a phrase that came into being in the late 1970s, appears to be the more politically correct term to use and the preferred choice of many cross-dressers.

Denzil/Damara. 'I didn't start cross-dressing until I was in my mid-twenties, long after I had joined the army. I had always held a fascination about what it must be like to be a biological woman. Then one day my curiosity got the better of me and I sought out some female knickers and tights, pleasantly discovering instant sexual arousal the moment I touched their tender silky texture. I was like a teenage boy who had discovered masturbation for the first time. I simply couldn't stop wanking. From then onwards, I wore panties whenever I could. Even during active service, I slyly managed to wear them under my combat gear. After I left the army, I threw out all of my male underwear and from then onwards have always worn women's underwear because I find them so comfortable and sensual.'

It is estimated that 3 out of every 100 males cross-dress. Cross-dressers are predominately male, heterosexual and married with families. They come from all walks of life including the police force and the construction industry. They usually start cross-dressing during puberty. Some will have sexual fantasies about being female whilst enjoying their male gender identity, as well as fully enjoying the benefits of their male bodies and genitalia. Ultimately, they have no desire to change their sex. Their motivation is distinctly different from that of a trans woman. Their brains are male and are in congruence with their male bodies. They view their bodies as being appropriate to their gender identity.

Keith/Kelly. 'It is not just panties; female clothing on the whole is far more comfortable than men's. I saw a young woman get on the train recently wearing a loose dress with just a bra and panties underneath. I was so envious of her because she looked so comfortable. There I was in jeans, shirt and jumper and I felt smothered. I wondered how good it would be for me to venture out in public like that woman on a summer's day, dressed as she was and looking as if she didn't have a care in the world.'

There are few female cross-dressers. They tend to keep low profiles and there are hardly any regular support networks available for them to meet other females who like wearing men's clothing. It is sometimes argued that females have less reason to cross-dress because society is far more accepting about female clothing standards: women can wear masculine clothing or actual male attire, for example a man's suit, without attracting much attention, as it can be passed off as a fashion statement.

Another major difference between male and female cross-dressers is the underlying motivation to cross-dress. I know of no suggestion that females masturbate during puberty by wearing men's underwear, or, during adulthood, wearing men's clothing to elicit sexual arousal or dressing up as a fetish.

The following extracts feature older men who have cross-dressed for several decades. These enlightening facets of life feature some who openly live as cross-dressers within a marriage, to those facing old age and death, as well as some who share optimistic views of how cross-dressers should be treated in the world.

Ryan/Rachel. 'We live in a post-modern world. We have legislation on our side. We have society on our side. Never has there been a point in time when cross-dressers were freer than they are presently.

I am a male nurse by profession. Some days I don't wear female clothes, mainly because I am too exhausted by the time I get home from work. But I always sleep in a nightie. God, I would be horrified if you asked me to wear a pair of men's pyjamas! Admittedly, cross-dressing was exhilarating and a bit of a turn on when I first started many, many years ago, but those moments have passed. To me it is the external pleasures that now bring me satisfaction. I enjoy social contact and companionship with other like-minded cross-dressers, but this is always in private settings. I wouldn't have the courage or the desire to walk down the street in a dress.

Do I pass as a woman when dressed? No man is happy with the way they look when dressed as a woman. They are always nervous in the company of others, wondering if they have done enough to pass. Yes, envy has its place when I see others who I feel are more convincingly dressed than I am. But when I am in the company of my close friends then these thoughts and fears abate, resulting in me feeling totally relaxed and at ease with myself. These are cherished moments.

Although most cross-dressers are perfectly happy dressing up as much or as little as they desire, there are some men who take their practice a little more seriously. It is not unknown for some men to take low grade hormones that they have bought on the internet, or they have electrolysis. Then there are those who have chest enhancement surgery, which they conceal when in male mode.

For me personally, it is nonsense when people refer to their alter-ego as if they were a person split in two. I fear their boundaries and perceptions have become blurred. It is as if they think they are split in two and that you need to treat each part differently to the other. But I consider everybody to be just one person. I accept there are many parts to me but at the end of the day these parts merge together into one. I know that when I cross-dress I am not so different to how I am when I am dressed as a man. I think the same, my opinions don't vary and ultimately what people are getting is the real me. I don't want them to treat me differently as if I was another person.

Maybe I have developed this confidence through time and wisdom. Maybe as I grow older my attitude has changed towards life and my relationship with the world and its people. Opinions are not always rigid and fixed. Cross-dressing is just a part of me, not some other foreign entity that is far removed from my normal everyday life and not separate from me as a whole. It simply is what it is and something that I have always very much enjoyed doing for all of my adult life.'

Peter/Petra. 'I hate the term "transvestite" because it conjures up naughty things. Okay, I have one or two fetishes, like dressing up in a maid's costume. I have a favourite leather PVC outfit that I sometimes slip into before I do some housework. My wife loves this because I do all the polishing and hoovering!

Cross-dressing for me has absolutely nothing to do with sex. I have cross-dressed for over 30 years and although I used to get aroused in the early days, there was nothing sexual about the experience, mainly it was one of feeling sensual from the different fabrics in women's clothing that are very different to men's. Over time, I discovered how my psyche alters every time I change into women's clothing. It feels like I am no longer a bloke but instead I feel feminine, softer and gentler for that period of time until I change back into my male clothes.

I have absolutely no idea what it really is that causes cross-dressing. There are lots of theories. I once read somewhere that a large majority of men feel that they would like to cross-dress but never get around to actually doing so. There are those who recognise that it is men who have stressful jobs, like truck drivers, paramedics, policemen and ex-army officers who cross-dress because it is between the two extremes. The thing about cross-dressing is the macho side switches off and the feminine side emerges, making one able to instantly relax. However, having said that, I am an accountant and have never felt stressed. I could hypothesise about my own reason for cross-dressing though. My father was away in the forces and I was brought up alone by my mother. I became fascinated with her knickers and tights from an early age and it manifested itself from there. It is just something I have always done since childhood and something that feels natural to me. For the past 20 years, I have built up a wardrobe of my own clothes and I'm pleased that I have more clothes and shoes now than my wife.

I remember my father being very ill in intensive care and me blaming myself for attracting bad karma. Although my father didn't know my secret, a voice at the back of my head said, "Someone doesn't like you cross-dressing." So I stopped and got rid of all my clothes. Then my father died and I sank into a deep depression. I loved my father and missed him dearly, but the truth is I also loved my dresses and missed them more. It felt like a part of me was missing so I started to buy women's clothes again and was instantly freed from my depression.

My wife was very surprised when I told her about my cross-dressing and the name I had chosen for my alter-ego. But it was my late mother-in-law who came to my rescue. She asked my wife, "Do you love him?" Thankfully, my wife replied, "Yes, of course I do." We have stayed together and I can genuinely say that we both enormously love and respect each other. When my daughter found out, she was upset, but these days she has a far more relaxed approach to me and hardly bats an eyelid when she sees me in a dress.

The strangest thing is that when I dress as a woman, my mannerisms change. So does my body language, as well as the way I stand and the way I walk. When I am in a group of other cross-dressers, the furthest thing on my mind is football, rugby or cricket. Instead, we talk freely about hair, make-up, clothes. I remember once being in the throes of one of these conversations when I suddenly thought, "Jesus, we are all blokes!"'

Barry/Bethany. 'I got rid of all my clothes. I am an old man now and didn't want my relatives to find them after I died. They have no idea that I cross-dressed for 35 years, no inkling at all. I lived a double life. I offered to give my clothes to other men in my social group, but they declined. I guess the thing about cross-dressers is that they all have their own taste in clothes and usually have an abundance of their own style.

I spent over 35 years in the Royal Navy as an engineer. Here, I had to be ultra-masculine because in those days even if you wore aftershave, you were called gay. I had a girlfriend who let me down, resulting in me never getting married because I was unable to ever trust another woman. My fascination with cross-dressing started with women's sandals and it is a fascination that still lingers with me. These days the sandals are more unisex than anything else. I have about 20 pairs. The first thing I have always done when I see a beautiful woman is to look at her feet. Some might say I have a fetish for footwear, but I have big feet – size ten and wide – and can only find comfort in sandals. The problem with men's sandals is that they have always been so plain and dull, while women's are prettier and more colourful.

I adore Asian clothing, especially saris as they are so comfortable to wear, because I find them so striking, colourful and the silky fabric is so sensual to touch. Nothing gave me more pleasure than to slip into one after having a bath when I got home from a hard day's work. I used to refer to them as my loungers which I wore coupled with a pretty pair of brightly coloured muse sandals. I had little interest in make-up, although I occasionally wore lipstick.

I once told a doctor that I liked women's clothes. He referred me to a psychiatrist who asked me to describe my feelings. I said to him, "It's like being in a room surrounded by beautiful women who are all smoking and you desperately want to light a cigarette but you are forbidden. In your pocket you have the finest packet of cigarettes and gold lighter but you are not allowed to touch them." I finished the sentence off by asking him how this would make him feel. He did not answer, although he reassured me that there was nothing wrong with me and that I did not need treatment. I knew myself that there was nothing wrong with me but I guess it was nice to get confirmation. The simple truth is, whether you are a transvestite or a cross-dresser, it is a harmless practice. Nobody gets hurt in the process.'

Wayne/Wendy. 'My social skills have never been great, and that was a contributing factor to the doomed relationships I had during my twenties and thirties and partially because none of my girlfriends could match my mother's qualities – tall, elegant and well-dressed. Our arguments about what they wore and how they looked ended whatever future we may have had.

Once you start dressing, your sexual tastes change. You develop new ones because you create a new identity. It is like becoming a new person. For me, I have many memories of my failures as a man, but when I dress as a woman these failures no longer exist. I am not attracted to gay men, especially gay men who are effeminate. My father was a retired army officer who was always impeccably well-dressed. I have always liked seeing men who, like my father, wear smart suits and ties. I deplore seeing men walking around the streets in beach wear or shorts and flip-flops, because it is such a turn-off. I consider myself bisexual because I have had six relationships with men but only when dressed in my female clothing. It is always my alter-ego that has sex with these men and not me.

Dressing in women's clothing was sensual in the early days, but after I had done it for a while the excitement wore off. It became part of a lifestyle. When I am at home, I dress mainly as a woman, although most of the time you can find me in just a pair of panties and a top. If I need to pop out to the supermarket, I usually just put on a pair of my male jeans and a jumper. It's easier that way because otherwise, putting on make-up and a wig can take up to 45 minutes. I don't feel revulsion towards my male clothes because deep down I don't have any deep-rooted hatred towards my masculinity. I accept I am a man and am comfortable with my gender. Overall, the clothing in my wardrobe is 60 per cent female and 40 per cent male.

Apart from never being able to find a woman who exuded my mother's style and elegance, I have no idea why I cross-dress. It's much easier to analyse other men and not one's self. I know of some men who have complained that their wives turned out to be too masculine in their mannerisms and dressing habits, which left them feeling dissatisfied. I doubt if any man marries a woman wanting his wife to be more masculine than he is. In cases like this, men crave a feminine aura and if they are not receiving it from their wives, they take on a role reversal and start to create the femininity they crave – or they leave. Those who start cross-dressing discover a sexual eroticism that pleasantly surprises them. It brings satisfaction, enjoyment and creates something vigorous in their lives that may have been otherwise missing.

Things will change, though. I am confident that in 20 years' time, or maybe even less, cross-dressers will be able to be more open about themselves because society will be far more tolerant. I can see the day coming when men and women will be able to pick and choose how they present at work – be it cross-dressing in the opposite gender, or alternating between both gender expressions – with each person feeling respected for their masculine and feminine presentations.'

Cross-dressers find comfort in dressing in women's clothes as they find it's relaxing and brings temporary freedom from the pressures of being male. It is a form of expression that is personal to them. However, there is a distinct difference between a cross-dresser and a trans woman. Trans women believe they have a right to dress in female clothing because they are *female.* They have female brains. Male cross-dressers will invariably never have had any thoughts of wanting to become women. They will never have experienced gender dysphoria or dislike of their body. Basically, they will never feel this incongruence between their brain and gender assigned to them at birth and are happy retaining their birth identity in their everyday lives which is devoid of gender dysphoria stress.

Some trans people believe that cross-dressers lessen the integrity of trans women and accuse them of dressing as women for a thrill-seeking pleasure or for some sort of sexual gratification. It must be noted though that there are some trans women who have experimented with cross-dressing earlier in their journey to see if this would help alleviate mental anguish; but once they realised that it didn't fulfil their inner feelings they proceeded to the transitioning route so as to live full-time in their new gender.

A considerable number of cisgender women are comfortable with men who cross-dress, although they often dismiss it with humour. Non-cross-dressing men, though, often feel it challenges their masculinity and are hostile and discriminatory as a result. There is also much homophobia attached to this because of a lack of understanding on the subject. There are some macho men who persistently like to boast when they are with each other about cars, wives and lovers, so dropping the subject of cross-dressing into this hard world of machoism is difficult. There are other men who would like to experiment but reject the idea after they start wondering if they are gay by showing an interest in female clothing.

What is common amongst cross-dressers is that nearly all of them will have experienced at least one purge at some time or other in their cross-dressing lives, trying to suppress their desires by throwing away all their feminine attire. When a person purges they stop cross-dressing because they are overcome with feelings

of shame or guilt. It is not unusual for people to clear out
their clothes, wigs and jewellery, believing that once they
get rid of these, they will be free from the compulsion to
cross-dress ever again. But the purge usually proves to be
short-lived because it does not relieve the inner conflict
going on within the person and results in them buying
new clothes and starting all over again.

The next set of extracts feature younger cross-
dressing men and outlines some of the difficulties they
often face in keeping balance in their daily lives. Again,
the alter-ego is mentioned and the importance that is
placed on this by some when referring to sex. Purging
is featured too, but the overriding factor is the degree
of normality that these men view their cross-dressing,
to the point it has become an ingrained, non-negotiable
part of who they are.

Des/Denise. 'There was something about Boy George
and Culture Club that resonated with me. I said to
myself, "Well, if he can do it, so can I." A fascination
with female clothing has always flooded my mind,
but when I was younger I couldn't rationalise my
thoughts. I hadn't the confidence to tell anybody
how I was feeling and never plucked up enough
courage to be seen dressed in public. I was timid and
shy and grew up always feeling different. I wasn't
gay and neither did I have a trans brain. I have never
been into girls and have never had a relationship. Sex
has never mattered to me.

In my late teens I started experimenting with shoes
and clothes, mainly my mother's, and sometimes I
sneaked a few things out of my sister's wardrobe to
try on. I have a great relationship with my mother.

She knows me and accepts me fully. One day she asked if she could see me dressed as Denise. I did as she requested and seeing me dressed did not faze her. It had the opposite effect on my stepfather who, I knew by the expression on his face, did not like what he saw. He didn't speak to me for two days afterwards.

My sister is great too. She often refers to me as a brother and sister all rolled into one. She even sometimes gives me her opinion or advice on what to wear if I am going out with some of my cross-dressing friends.

Up until a few years ago, I used to get all my clothes from mail order catalogues and then from the internet, but these days I buy them in shops. Even with this my sense of confidence has increased, because not so long ago I was unable to walk into a shop without someone accompanying me.

I like the girly side of myself and veer towards this more and more as I get older. I am 30 now. I have slowly abandoned the macho things I liked earlier in my life. I changed from a job in engineering and trained to be a hairdresser. I dropped listening to heavy metal music and switched to jazz. In female clothing, I have mannerisms and expressions that make me feel more at ease with myself. This lessens my stress and also my anxieties around others. I am constantly scrutinising females, not in a salacious or freaky type of way but rather I enjoy learning from observing their posture and the way they walk. If I see some mannerism in a woman that I particularly admire, I try to copy it. I veer towards women who are femme and ladylike.'

Connor/Concetta. 'On one level, the intrigue for many cross-dressers is dressing as a woman and taking this to a level when they hope to convincingly pass as one. Female clothes for men are extremely erotic – texture and a tight fit brings arousal to lots of men. Stockings and suspenders bring their fair share of thrills too. For me, my sexual buzz begins from the moment that I start taking clothes out of my wardrobe. For the first 20 minutes while I'm getting dressing I get turned on. The sensation of an internal erection is present. I know of men who say their scrotum retracts completely when they get a sensation of this kind.

A lot of men tend to present to the world in male macho mode – both at work and in the family home. This can be hard because they crave the next opportunity that they'll be able to dress in female clothes. Until this moment arrives, which can sometimes be days or even weeks, they rely in the meantime on a comfort blanket. This can be something as simple as wearing a pair of knickers or popping some mascara in their pocket.

I am Jewish and the thought of my family finding out absolutely terrifies me. I wouldn't be able to cope with the rejection. I am extremely careful about not being caught out. My wardrobe is always locked at home just in case my mother or another member of my family visits or stays overnight. In summertime, I never shave my arms or legs because this too would be a giveaway.

I believe every cross-dresser on the planet experiences at least three purges during their lifetime. When I have these thoughts, I always consider what

I am doing is something perverse and goes against the norms of society. But anytime I have purged, I have been deeply upset after dropping off my clothes to a charity shop. Instead of feeling the relief of no longer having to live a double life, thoughts of me throwing away a part of me blitz my mind, and on the two occasions I have purged, the regret of doing so outweighed any guilt or shame. I have always gone back to cross-dressing after things had settled down.

Although I describe myself as bisexual, I have never slept with another man. I am particularly drawn to elegant women, particularly those that wear lots of make-up and have big hair like the late Amy Winehouse. I fantasise about sleeping with women like this and have been lucky to have had conquests matching this description. In instances like this, I do not see myself as a man who is sleeping with a woman. Neither do I consider myself a lesbian during these encounters. During sexual intercourse, I take on the passive role by insisting the woman gets on top of me.'

Victor/Victoria. 'I wear female clothes because I like them more than men's. When I was around the age of ten, I remember becoming envious of my female cousins. I thought their clothes were so much more colourful and comfortable than the ones I was made to wear. Every time I touched their clothes, I recall finding them soft and tender.

I often wonder how we survived without the internet. Before this many people were sitting at home, lonely and wondering if we were the only ones in the world that dressed in women's clothes.

Many people will have questioned if they were weird or freaks or some other abnormality in society. But even in today's knowledgeable world, there needs to be much more education in society about cross-dressers and their lives – likewise amongst cross-dressers themselves. Presently, there is little written on the subject. I would love to find out more about the history of cross-dressers from the 18th century to the present day because I imagine this would reveal many fascinating facts about what people have gone through down the years to express this side of their lives.

A few of my friends know that I cross-dress but I have never come out to my family. I have a relative who is trans and during the time of her transition from male to female, I listened to them scream slurs and prejudices, rather ignorantly linking it to paedophilia and homosexuality. I feel if I told them, I too would become subject to a barrage of ignorance and discrimination. They would probably think of me as gay or say I was a pervert or a weirdo.

We are not freaks. We are ordinary people. We just have a different part of us that other people don't have. Personally, I feel being a cross-dresser has made me a much more rounded person. I see the world differently because it has taught me more about women than I would have otherwise known. I have a better understanding of how they are treated, how they think and what they desire. This understanding wasn't entirely gained by direct experience but through shared stories from other cross-dressers. But I do constantly observe the world around me all the time that non-cross-dressers may not notice. I take notice of window displays and often wonder when I see a gorgeous dress what I would look like wearing it. I doubt if a male non-cross-dresser would even notice the window, let alone realise the beauty of the dress or wonder if the shop had it in their size. The matter of dress size is always a concern for me because I am a large lady.'

Philip/Pamela. 'I find that some men go to great lengths to conceal their cross-dressing, especially married men. I remember once going to a support gathering and having to share a room with another person. He walked in with two battered-looking suitcases and two black bin liners. I wondered why he had taken so much luggage. It turned out that he had to hide all his clothes from his wife in a secret hiding place in the garage and hadn't had an opportunity to sort through them before he left. The clothes in the bin liners were all bundled up and full of creases. Likewise for the clothes in the suitcases. My God, the stench of mustiness and body odour stank the room. He explained that he was never able to wash any of his clothes at home in case his wife discovered his secret. I spent some of the weekend helping him wash and dry his clothes on the balcony to our room. But at least we saw the funny side to it and had a good laugh. He left at the end of the weekend with his laundry complete. It made me realise how lucky I am to be single and carefree, without having the added stress of a partner who doesn't know the real me.

Although I have never told my parents that I cross-dress, I am confident that they know, which I am totally fine about. My mother always waters my plants when I'm away on holiday. Last year, I had a new bathroom fitted before I went away. She told me after I returned home that she went into the house to see the bathroom and commented on how lovely she thought it was. I don't hide things in my house and if my mother had opened my bathroom cabinet she would have found it bulging with mascara, foundation, lipsticks, perfume and so on. If she had ventured into my bedroom and opened my wardrobe, she would see the most amazing collection of dresses, all hung up and mingled in with my male clothing and work uniform. I find it inconceivable that she wouldn't have taken a peep in my absence.

When I hear people talk about their alter-ego, I find their boundaries are blurred. I am suspicious and feel it is a fallacy, with some men taking it to the extreme. Once I heard a fellow cross-dresser say that when he is driving to his support group dressed in female clothes that he is a much more careful and considerate driver than when he is in male mode. Another one said he likes to keep his female and male clothes in separate wardrobes because he likes to see himself as two separate people. Others claim to be happily married but yet they sleep with men when cross-dressed and later claim that it wasn't their married male part of themselves that had sex, rather their single female alter-ego. They don't see it as cheating but I very much doubt if there are many people outside the world of cross-dressing that wouldn't see this for what it really is. These men are merely fooling themselves by thinking that their reality is split in two. A person only has one mind and the part of the mind that dictates a motivation to cross-dress is not so unlike the remainder of the mind. Both sides merge together. For me, I don't want these two parts of myself to be seen as different components.'

As is clear from the last set of extracts, there is often a strong element of secrecy around being a cross-dresser, with many living double lives. Shame and embarrassment prevail over the truth and, at best, only a handful of people will be privy to the true reality. Cross-dressers accept this as part of their lives because it is a method that works for them. Undoubtedly, their greatest fear is discrimination and hostility if they were to be open about their lives.

Michael/Mary. 'It's the secrecy bit that is a killer. When a wife finds out, she instantly asks "Why didn't you tell me this before?" Then she wonders, "What will we tell the children? What if the neighbours find out?" This is quickly followed by more personal internalising as she questions, "What else has he been up to? Is he gay? Does he have sex with other men?" The wives even question their own sexuality and wonder whether they are lesbian if they are married to a man who dresses as a woman. These marriages either survive or they don't. Some couples stay together for the sake of their children or for financial security or some other dependency but live unhappy lives. Some might question if it is better for a wife not to know that her husband cross-dresses and for all concerned to remain none the wiser.'

When somebody asks if there is a cure for being a cross-dresser, or indeed any of the other trans identities, the sensible answer must be *Should there be one?* The propensity to try and cure people hails from the heteronormativity culture that comes with the belief that people fall into two genders and that anything that deviates from this norm is an aberration that needs to be cured. Gay people too have had these cure myths thrust upon them, which are both meaningless and insulting. Ultimately, they don't work. They can't work because they are trying to cure something that is not a problem, although societal values may have convinced the person otherwise. However, the irony of trying to cure something that is normal is in itself an abnormality.

Daly/Donna. 'My wife fell pregnant. I remember saying to myself, "Oh Lord, I am about to become a father, I must cure myself of this affliction." I went to my GP and told him I liked dressing in women's clothes. "Oh, you are a transvestite", he said. "If you are serious about getting cured, I will refer you to a psychiatrist." I hated the sound of that. This was in the late '50s. I hadn't a clue what transvestite meant and neither had my wife. We looked it up in the dictionary. It read: A form of sexual deviant behaviour – a sexual perversion. My wife instantly thought that I was a sex pervert. So did I.

There was no question then of me not going to see the psychiatrist. My wife insisted on it. I went every three weeks for a six-month period. I'd change into my dress and put on some make-up. The psychiatrist would give me an injection in the buttocks, which after a few minutes would start the vomiting. While I was being sick, he would subject me to a barrage of abuse that lasted ten minutes or so. He'd say things like, "You dirty, silly pervert! You loathsome specimen of mankind! Why on earth do you think you are a woman? You have got to stop this crazy idea once and for all!" The whole episode was madness from start to finish. Of course, it didn't cure me. Why would it? You can't change who you are by these foolish means. Thank God these methods are no longer used, but can you imagine the emotional upset this was likely to have caused to other emotionally vulnerable people whose confidence and self-esteem were already at a low ebb.'

CHAPTER SEVEN

SEX AND SEXUALITY

Regina, trans woman. 'Looking in the mirror made me ask questions of myself – the basics of who and what I was. I was a man who had always felt different and had now discovered, after years of soul searching, that the moment had arrived. For me to have any true contentment and freedom of mind, the only answer was to become a woman. There was no doubt about this, and deep down perhaps there never was, but for the first time I began to doubt my sexuality. Was I gay or bisexual – or was I a heterosexual woman who wanted to have sex with a man? I was confused. What people don't realise is that transsexuals and sexuality are not opposite sides of the coin. They aren't even the same currency.'

Research

There has been little research into the subject of sexuality in relation to trans people. Most of the work related to this topic is based on anecdotal evidence and shared general experiences and this chapter captures the opinions of trans people whom I interviewed. Their views capture a whole gambit of human sexuality and what it means to connect and be attracted, both physically and emotionally, to another person, often without having to remain within the confines of a sexual orientation label. Trans people, most often trans women, are fetishised by some cisgender people and this results in a demand for pornography featuring trans people. Many trans people consider this an offensive and upsetting dehumanising distortion of their identities and bodies. It also means trans people are placed at increased risk of experiencing unwanted sexual propositions, harassment and even sexual assault.

Sexual orientation

It is generally considered that with trans people, sexual orientation is based on the current gender. Changing body doesn't necessarily mean changing sexuality. A person's fundamental sexual orientation usually does not change after an individual's transition, irrespective of whether they have any hormones or surgery or neither of these. However, it is important to take into consideration how this is interpreted – for example, a trans woman who previously presented as heterosexual may still pursue relationships with women after transitioning, although afterwards she may identify as lesbian.

Felix, trans man. 'You have to look at people and step back. Society is too hung up on labels. In my opinion trans people retain the same attraction to the sex they were attracted to before they transitioned, although this manifests itself differently once the person changes gender and can result in the person being re-labelled gay or heterosexual depending on the circumstances. In my case, I have always been attracted to women and after I transitioned to male, society has viewed me as heterosexual, although beforehand I was viewed as a lesbian.'

Trans people have the same range of sexual orientation as cisgender people and therefore may describe themselves as lesbian, gay, bisexual, straight ot use other similar terms. A survey carried out by Trans Equality Network Ireland *Speaking from the Margins: Trans Mental Health and Wellbeing in Ireland* (McNeil *et al.* 2013) discovered that out of 107 trans people interviewed, 30 per cent stated that they were bisexual, 23 per cent heterosexual, 17 per cent lesbian and 7 per cent gay.

Identity and interpretation

A trans woman who has not had genital reassignment surgery may have relationships with men and view these as straight encounters. Alternatively, she could have relationships with women and view herself as lesbian – or she could be bisexual.

People who have transitioned can find it difficult to attract suitable partners. Some of them feel invisible afterwards, owing to the rejection they encounter from people their own age who cannot cope with the idea of them being potential lovers. Others notice a difference in the way they perceived themselves prior to transitioning, in the sense that they did not encounter problems in sexual relationships, but following transitioning struggle to find sexual partners who are interested in them as the person they are. They come into contact with people who want them to have a sexual organ that they no longer have or who seek them for the novelty of the sexual organ they now have, resulting in a dysfunctional liaison or relationship from the outset.

For trans men metoidioplasty is often an acceptable alternative to phalloplasty, as the clitoris becomes a micro-phallus that can greatly enhance the sexual satisfaction of both the trans person and their partner. On the other hand a phalloplasty, which includes an internal prosthetic to enable erection, can contribute greatly to the physical and emotional satisfaction of the trans person and their partner during sexual intercourse. Trans women who have had a vaginoplasty can have satisfactory intercourse too, aided by lubrication. However, for many trans people and their partners such surgery is still very difficult to obtain, and most couples, whether heterosexual or gay, will find their own ways of developing their sexual relationship in a manner which redefines the trans person's birth genitals to match their new gender.

The following extracts illustrate how various trans men and women view their sexuality themselves, and how other people sometimes inflict their prejudice and interpretation of sexuality upon them.

Grayce, trans woman. 'Before transitioning, I disliked being interpreted as female. I was butch and awkward. I hated the way I sat, drank my tea and walked. Hormone therapy is a mysterious thing. Over the course of a couple of months I swapped being female and butch to being male and camp. There was another bonus too for me. Lesbian relationships – which were easy for me to form – were replaced with relationships with men. This was a distinct blessing because it made me realise how much I didn't really fancy women. I was left in no doubt where my true sexuality lay and for the very first time in my life I explored relationships and sex with vigour that I had never imagined possible.

I consider myself queer as opposed to being gay, but on the surface I appreciate that I will be perceived as a gay man who is in a relationship with another man. The reason I mention queer is because I am capable of sexual attraction to trans and non-binary men. Coming out to new partners is always tricky though, and at first it became a balancing act as to when to choose the right time to divulge my trans identity. I discovered it was best to tell them early into the relationship by saying something simple like, "Actually, I'm trans, are you okay with that?" I told my current partner early in the relationship and have now been in a civil partnership for six years.'

Darryl, trans man. 'I can honestly say that for the last 12 years I have been immensely happy living as a man. I have never fancied men and have always been sexually attracted to women. I don't feel the need, at this point in my life, to have genital surgery because I believe that, irrespective of genitals, a person can replicate any sexual practice.'

Luke, trans man. 'I am a gay man but not in a relationship. I have never been in a relationship since I transitioned. I suspect that other gay men will expect me to have certain body parts that I don't have as I have not had lower surgery. But I feel male in every other possible way. When I stand naked in front of a mirror, I see myself as the person I have always wanted to be. Perhaps, having phalloplasty would enhance my life but for now I feel complete without it. It is not a priority because I feel a body is only a shell we live in. It does not define us exclusively as human beings.

I love being the person that I am. I consider my life to be amazing. I have seen it from a different perspective. I have been on the most enlightening journey. I have got to know myself really well in the process. Overall, it has been a most liberating experience. I joke that I am post-gay and belong to a new frontier in male sexuality. I dislike the gay community sometimes, because a few of the most narrow-minded people I have ever met were from the gay community. The dominant tendency of gay men – which I do not feel part of – is to focus on what is in a person's pants. In my pants, I have a vagina. In fact, that is what can be found in the pants of most trans men.'

Rosie, trans woman. 'A lot of trans women find themselves in a similar situation to mine. I fully accept that I am a biological man who happens to be a female heterosexual. I have no sexual interest in women. My life comprises an outward role of a woman (I have not had reassignment surgery because I never felt the need) with my deepest inner need being completely fulfilled through the gender role of a woman, through which I have lived my life for the past 25 years.'

Harley, trans man. '"What's the story about your genitals?" is a question that I am most asked. There appears to be vulgar curiosity, especially amongst gay people who feel they have a right to ask these questions. Gay people love asking about sex and genitals – they haven't learned yet that such enquiries are unacceptable. I know sometimes that people can be curious and not necessarily in a mean way, but they find it odd when I refuse to answer. Gay people have often asked me, "Are you a top or bottom? Do you wear a strap-on? Can I see your genitals?" The cisgender world is also obsessed about sexual labels and genitals. They too need to learn to be more inhibited and appropriate. Take a hint if a trans person doesn't like talking about themselves in this way.'

Alfie, trans man. 'I have never found my genitalia to be a problem when having a relationship, whether with women or men, even before I had genital surgery and now after it. I have had many sexual relationships – more with women than men, but all on the whole very satisfactory relationships. Perhaps that is because I have spent a lot of time coming to terms with my body as well as my bisexuality. Straight women and gay men really don't mind what genitals you have so long as they fancy you and you are honest. And I work hard to ensure I don't let my masculinity slip – the reason being that it is my masculinity they are attracted to. If I let my female self into the bedroom, they would not be attracted to me. I also concentrate on what they would like, what would make them want to reach an orgasm, because once they are ready, they really don't mind doing to me whatever it is I would like to reach an orgasm.'

Heteroflexible

'Heteroflexible' is a modern term for people who primarily present as heterosexual but experiment in other types of relationships, simply meaning that although they consider themselves to be predominantly heterosexual they occasionally have sex with people of other genders. Being heteroflexible can sometimes be interpreted as pushing boundaries and moving away from what is considered conventional sexuality, because some of the sex involved is considered queer, but nevertheless this is a term that is becoming more freely used within the trans community. Trans people with new genitalia following reassignment surgery may also wish to experiment with their new sexual organs to see what satisfies them sexually.

Some trans people postpone having sex until they have had genital surgery because they feel any sex before this won't fully reflect how they see themselves sexually. Like all sexually active adults, trans men and women will experience the natural concerns about how potential partners will see them: will they be found physically attractive? Trans people in particular may experience embarrassment at the prospect of being seen naked.

It must be noted that a wide range of sexual experiences take place in the trans community, although there's not any indication of this being more or less than what is experienced by gay or heterosexual people. The extracts that follow show a variety of preferences and the experimentation that helps create personal preferences.

Evie, trans woman. 'For the first time in my life, I started fancying men. People thought this strange and accused me of lying about my sexuality before I transitioned, but this simply wasn't true. There were never moments of internal conflict or internalised homophobia. It was simply something that had never crossed my mind before. I'm heterosexual and have no interest in gay men. I have only ever been in love with one woman – my ex-wife. I have only known what it is like to have sex with one woman and this was my ex-wife. But this mainly consisted of me having oral sex with her. Penetration was mechanical – an afterthought – or something I did to finish the job. After pleasuring her, I would go inside her to ejaculate but this was never important to me. I still love women, and I suppose if I were to transition I would enter into a lesbian relationship. There were times in my marriage when I wanted my wife to make love to me. I would have been quite happy to be submissive. Perhaps, I've always had the psyche of a woman who wanted to make love to other women.'

Violet, trans woman. 'I consider myself a straight female. I am sexually attracted to men. Anyway, I don't think it is anybody's business what I have got down in my dress. What goes on in my bedroom is entirely my business. I remember being in a gay bar a few years ago with a few of my friends. There were some lesbians present with short cropped hair and lumberjack shirts. Here was I in the early stages of transitioning and wishing that my breasts were bigger. I laughed out loud at the irony of the situation when I saw that the lesbians had bound their chests and I said to my friends, "They are trying to get rid of what we want."'

Roger, trans man. 'Although I am pansexual, my first relationship in my late teens was with a very pretty heterosexual girl. I liked this because I was able to explore my masculinity in a way I was never able to do before. But ultimately, I choose the people to have sex with based on their personality, irrespective of whether they are male or female. If I feel connected to someone, I pursue a relationship. Over the years I have had liaisons with lesbians, gay men, heterosexual men and those who are gay curious and trans curious.'

Sex drive

Some trans women comment that their sex drives have lessened after hormones and/or genital surgery. Some trans people may find that sex is not as satisfying functionally if their arousal and sensation becomes problematic due to surgery complications. Some other trans women may abstain from sex if their libido drops during hormone therapy. They may describe themselves as asexual, meaning that they have no sexual desire. They may share companionship with other people but do not have sexual relations.

Lucy, trans woman. 'I don't have a sex drive and have never had sex as a woman. In terms of sexuality, I am not attracted to women but neither am I sexually attracted to men, although these days since I transitioned, I feel more comfortable in the presence of men than I have ever felt in my life. I like the respect I get from men as a woman. One part of me thinks that if I allowed a man to make love to me, this would be a tick box exercise to say

I had sex in my new body. On the other hand, if I met a man who I fell in love with, who knows what might happen? So, on that note, I am keeping my options open. One of my friends jokingly suggests dating and escort agencies, although the latter scares me. But companionship would be lovely – someone to rely on, to talk to about things and someone to go out with for dinner and to the theatre.'

Some trans men feel that their sexuality changes after they commence hormone therapy – for others it does not. Trans men who take testosterone often have a much higher sex drive than trans women who take oestrogen. To begin with, trans men may masturbate as much as teenagers do during puberty. Some may also seek out frequent sex because of their urges. However, some trans men experience such gender dysphoria that they have a low sex drive despite taking testosterone. The level of sex drive is personal to everyone before, during and after transition.

Finlay, trans man. 'I worry about the effects that having a phalloplasty may have on my girlfriend, who is bisexual. I question if I will cause stress for our relationship by being grumpy while in pain during the weeks of recovery that the multiple operations entail. Will the penis look good enough or could it end up looking off-putting? I have concerns that going through phalloplasty may not improve our sex life and may even actually have the reverse effect and alienate her. Could it split us up?

I face the dilemma of still wanting to resolve my remaining dysphoria about my genitals, but at the same time fearing the high risks of surgical complications which phalloplasty entails. I know I will have to be careful when making love to my girlfriend because to be too rough may damage the penis. There is also a high risk of infection which could result in me losing the penis, and I know that no matter how effective the surgery is, the erection device has a time span of between seven and ten years before it needs replacing.

My girlfriend and I love each other. She is very accepting of me. We have a diverse sex life, although I have a preference for using oral sex to give her orgasms. But I have a lingering dysphoria about my vagina which significantly reduces my sex drive. I still feel that it does not belong to my body and want rid of it. Despite the fears and risks that surround genital surgery, it may actually turn out to be really beneficial for me. There is one other option to free me from the dysphoria I feel about my genitals – to maybe have a vaginectomy. But if I opt for vaginectomy on its own, it could mean I can't get a phalloplasty later on.'

New beginnings

It can be very difficult for a trans person to know in advance what will work well in terms of sexual relationships once they are living in a different gender or have had various surgeries. Therefore, some trans people find aspects of their sexuality develop in surprising, unexpected ways. Others may find they need to experiment with different relationship dynamics and/or ways of having sex during and after transitioning.

Patsy, trans woman. 'Before transitioning, I played the role of the alpha man. I wanted to convince myself that I could be a man. I was into weightlifting and bodybuilding. Conforming led me to getting married and having children. But all along I was less attracted to women and more attracted to men. I've heard of so many men doing the most extraordinary things to escape the truth. Although my leaning was towards men, I didn't want gay sex: my brain also told me that I was a woman, and I wanted a man to make love to me. Now that I have transitioned and have had full reassignment surgery, I consider myself to be a heterosexual woman.'

Maureen, trans woman. 'You have to consider how men in society view trans women. Straight men who are attracted to trans women question their sexuality once they find out that the woman hasn't had genital reassignment surgery. "Are you gay?" becomes their burning question. Some walk away and others don't but those that continue with the relationship are either married men or those already with girlfriends. They don't like to be seen in public with trans women but instead will ask if they can come to their home for sex. Younger trans women don't have a problem with this but some of us older ones do because we feel it is demeaning.'

Increasingly, trans people are finding that their pre-transition partners remain with them during and after transition. Staying in a relationship with a trans person who is transitioning can cause a variety of challenges. These include having to navigate through physical and emotional changes to try to maintain a satisfying sex life. It can also include finding that others start making incorrect assumptions about your sexual orientation. Unfortunately, many countries still insist that any marriage or civil partnership between a couple must be ended through divorce before legal gender recognition is given.

Sometimes trans people decide to date within the trans community. When two trans people form a relationship, this can enable each to feel better understood and supported in regard to their gender identities. However, it can also place stress on the relationship if one partner has better success than the other in achieving the physical changes they desire, which undoubtedly leads to resentment and jealousy.

Non-binary people and sex

The non-binary people I interviewed commented on the need to be comfortable around potential partners before divulging their sexual needs, but many of them said they preferred to partner with other non-binary people because they find this easiest. Where both parties are non-binary, they are more likely to understand and respect the other's identity without the need to justify or go into an explanation about what they need to make the relationship work – both emotionally and sexually. Some of these relationships can be between non-binary people who were assigned the same gender at birth or the opposite gender.

Starr. 'I have been in relationships with trans men and women, and cisgender women, however I have never dated a cisgender man. While I am open to the idea,

I am concerned about how I would be perceived, given my female body and the foreign dynamics of a straight relationship – both emotionally and physically. In this sense, being gender-queer can be complicated. In my experience of relationships so far, it has been my relationships with trans individuals that have been the most complicated. The inner turmoil of transition, and the body dysphoria associated with being trans, can be seriously damaging to a relationship. As a gender-queer person, I don't have that baggage. That's not to say that every gender-queer person doesn't though.'

Abigail. 'I find it much easier to like women now I'm not trying to be one. I'm generally attracted to women and androgynous people. Occasionally I'm attracted to a man but I wouldn't get into a new relationship on that basis as I'm not able to sustain sexual attraction for any length of time, so it wouldn't be fair. My sexual preferences are also affected by my anatomical differences as I have much more satisfying sex with people who acknowledge and interact with my non-standard bits of equipment; non-binary people tend to be better in this regard as they don't have the same formulaic attitudes to sex as most men and women.'

Bayley. 'As I see it, among trans people in general there are a lot more pansexual/bisexual people than in wider society, I guess because we see how bodies and genders are not intrinsically connected, and as we see our and other people's bodies transition, our previously held notions about what makes people attractive can widen quite a lot. I consider myself queer. Most non-binary people I know also identify that way. I think that it's a bit difficult to define yourself as gay or straight because it really puts things in a binary way, even if you are usually only attracted to one type of organ or gender presentation. I'm sure some non-binary people identify as bisexual because people are seeing bisexual as less and less about binary gender. I've seen some non-binary people want to use words like "gynophilic" or something which centres them around being attracted to either masculinity or femininity or neither. It's hard to say.'

Some non-binary people feel resentment towards the cisgender community, who are unable or unwilling to accept that somebody views themselves as neither male nor female or who feel they are both genders, and the impact that this has on societal perceptions of sexual orientation and relationship options. Others feel that gay and lesbian people are no more accepting than straight people.

Toby. 'Sexuality is an unavoidable subject matter and a contentious one for non-binary people. The gay community are not always friendly or accepting of us. If I'm not in the same perceived gender as them, they will not view me as the gender that I am. Gay people and indeed cisgender people have never had to question their gender and some have never questioned their sexuality. Sometimes there is simply too big a gap in experiences to overcome – too many gaps of privilege. Therefore, I seek connection and love from within the trans community. It is here where I consider it safest.'

Cross-dressers and sex

Generally, the issue of sex and fetishism (when it comes to cross-dressers) is often wrongly linked to being gay because the majority of cross-dressers are heterosexual. However, homosexuality and bisexuality will feature in this group, as it does in any other group in society, although cross-dressers may sometimes be in denial about their sexuality. Some will say they only have sex with a man when dressed in their female persona, which, according to them, does not make them gay.

Jason/Jessica. 'I emulate being a woman first and foremost to free me from my distress. Some might call me confused but I know I am not attracted to men when I am in my daily role as a man. But the moment I put on women's clothing, it is as if I am transformed all over with my appearance, body and mind being taken over by another force, leaving me with no option other than to surrender to its will. Every time I'm dressed as a woman I long to feel a man's penis inside my body or I long to suck a man's penis. At these moments, I am not a man in my mind. I am a woman. After all, isn't it a woman's prerogative to suck a man's penis?'

Those who rely heavily on the alter-ego principle may temporarily consider themselves a heterosexual woman when they engage in sexual practices with men, and afterwards revert to being a heterosexual male in their everyday lives with wives or girlfriends. Whether this is just a case of internalised homophobia remains questionable. Here are some more examples of their attitudes around sex.

Reece/Ruby. 'Although sex is not important to me, I am beginning to realise that my efforts in dressing as Ruby have paid off. I dress well. I'm told I look convincing as a woman. I believe that I am an attractive looking man, so I think I have transferred this attractiveness into Ruby's appearance. Only the other day, a friend remarked to me that men must find me attractive when they see me dressed as Ruby. I wonder what I would say, if a young man, say someone aged 25 to 30, asked me out on a date. Who knows, I might accept. I think it is best that I keep my options open because to do otherwise might not be fair to Ruby.'

Karl/Kassandra. 'I don't have a partner at the moment but have had many liaisons over the years. Am I straight, or gay, or bisexual? The jury is still out deciding on that one. Personally, I don't see myself as gay and although I have had sex with men, I have only ever done so when in cross-dressing mode. Maybe I am bisexual because I've had girlfriends in my twenties and thirties but I never married. None of the men I've had sex with have ever seen me dressed as a man. When I've had sex with them, I have always kept my wig and bra on as well as my make-up. During bareback sex, I have always felt entirely a woman for those few minutes. I have always considered this a great and enjoyable experience because one of my fantasies was wondering what it was like for a biological woman to be penetrated. Having sex with a man is something I could never do as a man. During sex, I am always Kassandra and never Karl.'

Brandon/Beverley. 'It's nonsense if people think that cross-dressers walk around in a state of arousal all the time, in the same way that some people think we are all gay – or straight – if you believe what they write in magazines. The truth is some cross-dressers are gay, some are heterosexual and some are bisexual.'

Archie/Audrey. 'I consider myself bisexual. I was once in a gay relationship. My boyfriend knew beforehand that I was a cross-dresser and said he was fine about it, but when we moved in together, he constantly made fun of me whenever I dressed in one of my favourite dresses and continuously criticised my figure and make-up. My self-esteem plummeted. One day, after a blazing argument, I could no longer tolerate his cruel remarks and told him to leave. I am pleased to say I have never seen him since.'

Sexual health

Trans people often find that feelings of gender dysphoria and fear of transphobia make it difficult for them to discuss their genitals and sex life with healthcare professionals. Undergoing any examinations of their genitals can be even more distressing. This can make it particularly challenging for them to get sexual health advice and treatments. The need to take precautions and prevent HIV and sexually transmitted diseases equally applies to trans people as it does for anybody else.

There is great variety in trans people's sexual behaviour but regardless of the gender identities and sexual orientations of the people involved, any anal or vaginal penetration needs to be preceded by the same type of precautions against HIV and sexually transmitted diseases – that is, by ensuring dental dams or condoms are used if either partner has HIV, or has had unprotected sexual activity with a partner whose HIV status is unknown. An issue for trans men and people assigned female at birth taking testosterone is that it makes the skin around the vagina much thinner, which allows for cracks and bleeding, thus increasing the risk of HIV if the person engages in unprotected sex. Condoms should also be used on any prosthetic penis/dildo or other sex toys as HIV and other sexually transmitted diseases can be transferred via the surfaces of such objects.

Care needs to be taken not to start using surgically constructed genitals too quickly after surgery as this can lead to complications such as wound infection, prolapse of a new vagina or damage to a new penile erectile prosthetic. The advice of the surgeon should be sought and followed in regard to when it is safe to take part in particular sexual activities. Surgically constructed genitals, although they do not naturally produce lubrication or other fluids, can still transfer HIV and other sexually transmitted diseases, although the risk is greatly reduced.

If a trans woman or man has unprotected penetrative or oral sex with someone who is HIV positive, they must seek medical intervention within 72 hours and obtain post exposure prophylaxis medication, which counteracts against HIV developing. The side-effects of this include diarrhoea and/or nausea. Trans women who are HIV positive can find the combination of taking antiretroviral and hormone treatment at the same time places the body under great strain. It is also known that antiretrovirals may cause facial fat loss which will alter appearance.

CHAPTER EIGHT

HEALTH

Sue, non-binary. 'I always have anxiety about using medical services. There is always the fear new doctors will not accept me as real or will try and turn me into something that I am not. They always seem to use the wrong pronouns, with some openly refusing to use "they" to refer to me, stating that they feel it is a term for an object and not a person. They are also overly inquisitive about sexuality and sex lives.'

Trans people experience health issues that escape ordinary members of the population. Having surgery, sometimes multiple operations, can place great strain on the body, particularly for older trans people. They often have unique bodies which retain several biological internal organs belonging to their assigned gender at birth. There are diseases, such as cervical cancer and prostate cancer, which are particular to certain physical characteristics usually associated with women or with men. Therefore, trans people may have health concerns related to the gender they were assigned at birth rather than their gender identity. Becoming ill is additionally hindered by anxiety because the person may fear being treated with indignity by the medical profession.

Trevor, trans man. 'I am aware that I have a body that most medical professionals don't get. When it comes to health professionals, I always ask who I can go to who will understand my body: somebody who will understand my hormone treatment as a trans man and the surgery I've had, and indeed the surgery I have chosen not to have, that is, genital reconstruction. In some cases where health care professionals know little of trans issues, people feel cut adrift with their health care. For me personally, I would like to talk to a professional about the risks of me getting cancer but I don't know who I can go and speak to about this.'

Hormone treatment

Cross-sex hormone treatment is a lifelong process. Over several years, cross-sex hormone therapy and/or gender reassignment surgery will mean a trans person no longer has functioning organs which produce the hormones of their birth sex. A trans person does not usually reach a point where hormone therapy can be stopped, as without their cross-sex hormone therapy they will have no functioning hormonal base, and consequently will develop severe osteoporosis within a very few years.

In the early years, some effects of the treatment are reversible, for example, within the first two to three years of hormone therapy, a trans man may stop his testosterone treatment, ovulate and become pregnant, and a trans woman may stop her oestrogen treatment and be able again to ejaculate and produce fertile sperm. However, after several years, many effects of hormone therapy are not reversible, such as the breaking of a trans man's voice, or a trans woman's breast growth.

The treatment puts a trans person's body through puberty for a second time, often with profound effects both physically and emotionally. Every cell in the body becomes aware that a new substance has entered its space. Frequent medical check-ups are especially advisable at first, until the body adjusts to the treatment. Annual blood tests are recommended to check for any abnormalities in the person's major organs and circulation.

Buying hormone drugs from the internet is filled with dangers. They may not be genuine or they may be out of date, contaminated or mislabelled as an incorrect strength. Even if the medication is within date and accurately labelled, it could still be harmful since the person will usually not be medically monitored and may accidentally take too much or combine it dangerously with another drug. However, there are several reasons why people may end up taking the risk of self-medicating as opposed to the more legitimate route of having it professionally prescribed. Some are hesitant to engage in services and want to keep their transition as private as possible. Others are anxious to get started as quickly as possible and grow impatient with the often very long wait to be seen by a Gender Identity Clinic. Non-binary people may decide to self-medicate based on their assumption the Clinic will not understand their gender identity and will refuse them access to hormones.

Just like any other person taking regular medication, care with diet, exercise and lifestyle choices must be taken into consideration. A healthy lifestyle containing regular exercise, balanced diet and avoidance of illicit drugs and excessive alcohol is paramount for all trans people in general who take hormone therapy. Smoking is known to reduce feminising effects in trans women taking oestrogen. Hormone treatment is also known to impact on cholesterol levels, so it's particularly important to have a diet which bears this in mind and does not increase the risk of heart disease or stroke.

Physical health needs for trans women and people assigned male at birth (non-binary)

Before a doctor prescribes hormone treatment, they will enquire about the person's overall health, weight and obtain a full family history. In addition to taking oestrogen, some trans women might also be taking a hormone blocker (an anti-androgen) to stop the body producing testosterone. However, if they have had genital surgery, or have undergone an orchidectomy, this does not apply because, once the testicles are removed, the person will produce less testosterone.

A major fear whilst on hormone treatment, especially oestrogen, is deep vein thrombosis (DVT). In order to prevent blood clotting, trans women need to stop taking oestrogen before surgery, whether this is related to gender reassignment surgery or another kind of general surgery, including cosmetic procedures. The older the person, the greater the risks. Therefore, regular monitoring of circulation is needed to catch any problem before it escalates into a crisis.

Prostate cancer is always a concern that lingers in the minds of trans women over the age of 50, although the risk of getting this is no greater than for the cisgender male population and non-binary people assigned male at birth. The prostate does not get removed during reassignment surgery, therefore trans women and those assigned male at birth need to get this checked periodically. This is an area where trans women and those assigned male at birth often face humiliation, unless they have a considerate and compassionate doctor who appreciates the sensitivity of this problem – and likewise hospital staff if surgical intervention is needed.

Cerise, trans woman. 'As an older trans woman, I worry more about my health than younger people. I guess because of my age, the likelihood of me developing prostate cancer is higher. You hear horror stories about people with prostate problems having to get up to the toilet several times during the night and having a horrible feeling of still having a full bladder after they've been to the toilet. I hope this never happens to me.'

The issue of trans women having children post-transition is a contentious one. There are small percentages who seek to have their sperm frozen (although this is very expensive) if they are undecided about having children. However, they need to do this before they commence treatment because sperm production is affected afterwards and eventually stops.

Hormone treatment will eventually make a trans woman infertile. The length of time this takes varies from person to person, although there is some clinical evidence that shows that trans women can regain fertility after many years on oestrogen therapy (however, if a trans woman has their testicles removed, this renders them irreversibly infertile).

Physical health needs for trans men and people assigned female at birth (non-binary)

A condition called polycythaemia, which is an over-production of red blood cells, is something that occasionally occurs in trans men or non-binary people assigned female at birth taking testosterone that requires monitoring. This is not an issue encountered by trans people on oestrogen.

Trans men or people assigned female at birth who are on hormone therapy need blood tests to detect any altered liver function. Some people have trepidation towards this medical monitoring and are known to avoid going for tests because they fear, if the levels are not right, that the treatment might get withdrawn from them.

Trans people assigned female at birth may wear chest binders whilst awaiting chest surgery. The binders are sometimes tight and often result in tissue damage, as well as chest infections because they make breathing shallower. Just as prostate cancer is a worry for trans women and those assigned male at birth, breast cancer is equally a concern for trans men who were assigned female at birth. Even if trans men have both breasts removed in chest reconstruction, there is still a risk because they may have some breast tissue remaining, so attention should be given to any lumps and changes that occur. However, research is ongoing whether or not a trans woman's risk of breast cancer increases when she takes oestrogen and grows breast tissue.

Some trans men or people assigned female at birth will have their eggs stored in case they want to consider, after hormone treatment has started, surrogacy at some future stage. Like trans women and people assigned male at birth who have sperm stored, the numbers are low and they are usually younger trans people. For those who do this, much consideration is given to the decision in comparison to trans people who had children before transitioning. Circumstances are different in the sense that those with children were married or entered into typical relationships under pressure to conform to society, or did so as part of internalised transphobia, in the hope they would be cured from trans identities.

Although, hormone therapy will eventually make a trans man or person assigned female at birth infertile, they can get pregnant during the early stages of the treatment, before it takes effect. Those who do get pregnant will need to stop hormone treatment to protect the foetus. The ovaries which produce eggs start to atrophy within the first three years of a trans man taking a correct testosterone dosage. There are examples of trans men getting pregnant later, but it is clear that they have used testosterone intermittently and often at a very low dose.

Trans men or people assigned female at birth who have not had a hysterectomy will still have their cervix and will require smear tests every three years up until the age of 50 and every five years when they get older. Smear tests are a necessary part of life in the screening of cancer. It is recommended that trans men and people assigned female at birth with a cervix should be offered screening from their twenties, even if they are not sexually active.

The cervix is a common place to get cancer and very often this is related to human papilloma virus (HPV).

This virus can lead to abnormal tissue growth and other changes to cells within the cervix which can lead to cervical cancer. It can also be the cause of genital warts, the most common viral sexually transmitted infection in the UK. Younger trans men may have benefited from the HPV vaccination which has been provided in the UK to those assigned female at birth, at school, since 2008.

After some time on testosterone, and without penetration, the vagina can become smaller and less flexible making intimate tests more uncomfortable.

Perry, trans man. 'I treat that aspect of my body like a car part, like a motorist who goes to the garage to get their car serviced. I go for this test every three years. It's a part of life – an inconvenience – like getting a parking ticket. I don't fuss unduly about it. I ignore any unpleasant stares I get in the Clinic. In fact, they are fewer these days because I am upfront about my identity. I'm not ashamed any more. I think this comes across because the procedure is usually done in a matter-of-fact type of way and then it's over until the next time and I feel assured that I haven't neglected myself.'

Psychiatry

Trans people view psychiatry as both a blessing and a curse. However, nearly every trans person will have come to the attention of a psychiatrist at some point or other in their lives. The mental health system can often appear confusing and stigmatising for trans people, with many believing that obtaining a psychiatric diagnosis should not be a precondition to accessing health treatments and legal gender recognition. The World Health Organization categorises *gender identity disorders* under *mental and behavioural disorders*, although currently there are proposals to remove gender identity related conditions from the mental health categories. The real issue is where treatment will be based, and whether it will continue being provided through Gender Identity Clinics based in psychiatric units. Furthermore, it is now reviewing that categorisation and will probably amend it to *gender incongruence*, which hopefully will pave the way towards declassification from psychiatric diagnostic manuals.

Grant, trans man. 'Being trans is not a mental illness any more than cancer is, or having a missing limb. Mental health has no bearing on being trans, thus anyone needing better mental health should follow the same path anyone else from society would follow, as it is not a related issue. I have a network of hundreds of trans people and all of them are strong-willed and have their heads screwed on better than most non-trans people. Indeed I know more non-trans people with mental health concerns/issues than I do trans people. There is nothing wrong with our minds: the problem lies in our bodies.

There is growing evidence now that being trans is a purely genetic physical issue and has nothing to do with the mind. Certain genes and combinations of genes can result in the formation of brain development counter to what the body has developed into, thus causing the problem. Thus the brain/mind is correct, so the body that must be changed to bring the two into harmony.'

Psychiatry views trans identities as a mental disorder and often treats trans people with scepticism. Trans people complain about the lack of time spent with them during their appointments, which is sometimes as little as ten minutes. Given the amount of stress and anxiety that trans people endure when coming to terms with their gender identity, many feel more time and more counselling needs to be offered. The mood changes as a result of hormone therapy often get little recognition.

Patrick, trans man. 'My gender identity was treated as a symptom of a mental health issue rather than my genuine identity. People's mental health improves significantly as a result of transitioning. Simply, there is less stress, less anxiety and the shift towards being your true self dispels the dominant mental torture that would otherwise have become deep-rooted.'

Self-harming behaviour and suicidal ideation

There are several reasons for self-harming behaviour including family difficulties such as a breakdown in relationships – which may result in trans people who are parents losing contact with their children. It may stem from a person's gender dysphoria as well as the frustration of waiting for gender reassignment treatment. It could evolve from loss of employment or reduced income as well as general feelings of guilt, shame or inadequacy and self-hatred towards their situation. Stress associated with social change during early transition may increase the risk of self-harm. Starting oestrogen may place trans women or other trans people taking oestrogen at risk of mood swings while their bodies get used to new hormone levels. Some people consider self-harming as an acceptable way to express and alleviate their distress.

Jerome, trans man. 'I have a self-harming history going back to when I was 17. It became a way of coping with my frustration and distress about having a female body. I questioned if I was a lesbian but something felt wrong. I didn't like being a girl. I didn't like my genitals. A voice in my head asked, "Am I a freak?" It was not until I came into contact with a youth worker who was a trans guy that I realised that I was too. It made perfect sense. A year later I told my mum but she wasn't happy about it. Thankfully, it did not prevent me from seeking help from the GIC. After a couple of years of waiting, I was approved to start taking testosterone, followed by chest reconstruction surgery and a hysterectomy. There were never any regrets. The burden had lifted. My body became more congruent to how I felt about myself.'

Edward, trans man. 'My emotional wellbeing was hugely affected by my parents' attitude when I came out as trans. They kicked me out of the house and I had to go and live with an aunt for my final year at secondary school. I wondered if they did not love me enough to accept me. I self-harmed as a result by making cuts to my arms. My self-worth was at a low ebb and I was very depressed. I also developed eczema.

  When I started on testosterone I had to deal with internalised transphobia. I still hated my body at that time and became obsessed at looking at young cisgender men. I was jealous that their voices were deeper than mine, that their bodies looked better, that they had bigger muscles and so on. I learned to like myself and after I went to Florida and had chest reconstruction, my self-belief began to improve. The youth service that I was part of also provided opportunities for me to develop better confidence and hope. Things are much better now and I haven't self-harmed in over a year.'

The most common method of self-harm for trans people is cutting. Self-harm is often linked to distress about physical characteristics which are incongruent with the person's self-defined gender identity and are mainly prevalent in pre-transition trans people. Receiving hormones and surgeries often ends the urge to self-harm. At the moment of acceptance of themselves, suicidal ideation decreases. A large percentage of trans people self-harm or express suicidal ideation because of the acute levels of prejudice they have to face from society. This is often coupled with not being taken seriously by medical professionals. A survey, *UK Trans Mental Health Study* (McNeil *et al.* 2012), recorded the following findings:

- 70 per cent of the participants were more satisfied with their lives since transitioning.

- 85 per cent were more satisfied with their bodies since undertaking hormone therapy.

- 90 per cent were more satisfied after undergoing genital surgery.

Suicide

Blossom, trans woman. 'I understand suicide. I
appreciate why some trans people contemplate it and
those who carry it out. You have got to remember
that up until a few decades ago hardly anybody knew
trans people existed. Then it was generally confused
as something associated to being gay. It was also
viewed as a mental disorder that needed psychiatric
intervention so it's hardly any wonder that so much
stigma and shame still seeps through. Coming out
as trans is unbelievably hard if you are married and
have children.

Suicides occur when people don't see a way
forward because of a lack of understanding from
family, friends and work colleagues. Verbal conflict
can be overwhelming. Isolation and depression take
hold. It is incredibly hard for the trans person to
make a decision about their lives that suits everybody.
In doing so, they put their own happiness and
future in jeopardy. If in the darkest hour the person
feels that they haven't the strength or willpower to
override the storm, then irrational thoughts take over.
They see their death as a bonus to all parties
involved, including themselves, as they imagine that
everybody's emotional pain, including their own,
will cease with their demise.'

The suicide attempt rate for young trans people is
very high, with over one third of transgender people
attempting suicide at least once. Research conducted
by PACE, a charity for LGBT people which works in

partnership with Brunel University in London, carried out a survey with over 2,000 people in England between 2010 and 2014. It found that 48 per cent of trans people under the age of 26 had attempted suicide. Thirty per cent said they had tried to commit suicide in the previous 12 months, while 59 per cent said that they had considered doing so at some point in their lives (Pace Charity 2014).

It was found that people who had experienced suicidal ideation or had attempted suicide had often faced rejection and both verbal and physical abuse within their families as well as suffering distress of abuse in their communities, in the workplace and in the media.

Aliyah, trans woman. 'I attempted suicide when I was 15. I felt alone and desperately unhappy and thought that I would for ever remain apart from everyone else. Then I told some friends what the problem was but they didn't seem that bothered or fazed by it. This gave me comfort. However, I remember bumping into a friend who I hadn't seen in years and who was part of my then group of friends. He seemed a little shocked that I was now a woman and when he recalled me telling him years ago that I was trans, he thought I was just trying to be different and hadn't taken me seriously. But what really saved me though was seeing a documentary on television about trans issues, and discovering that there were treatments available that would help me to live my life as a woman. What a relief this proved to be. For the first time ever, I began to realise that I wasn't weird.'

Tyler, trans man. 'When I was 13, I remember sitting with a hunting knife wanting to castrate myself, thinking, somehow, that it would fix things or, at least, the doctors would have to make me whole. I went to bed at night praying that an angel would change me in my sleep and I would awake in the right body. Unfortunately, that didn't happen.'

CHAPTER NINE

TRANSPHOBIA, DISCRIMINATION AND HATE CRIME

Transphobia is an intense dislike or prejudice against trans people. It is similar to homophobia. The word 'tranny' gets bantered around easily but this word is deeply offensive to trans people, the equivalent of calling a gay person a 'faggot'. Such terms are especially hurtful considering all the internal struggles, the heartache and everything else that trans people have to go through to be happy with their identity.

If you are trans and live in a country that is not LGBT friendly, it is fair to say that your life will be consumed with fear. But even in countries that are becoming increasingly accepting of LGB people, the trans community still face transphobia and discrimination that is disproportionate to other LGB people. One reason for this is that people are frightened about what they know little about or what has historically been given a poor name. Most societies these days comprise of different cultures, religions and ethnic groups, many of whom display greater intolerance towards difference in others.

Rosalynn, trans woman. 'Ethnic minority communities can be very insulting to trans people when they see them on the street. They do their utmost to call out obscenities. "Batty boy, you are a fake! You fool nobody!" are some of the things I have had said to me. They are ignorant and hypocritical because they fail to realise that people from within their own communities are trans and cross-dressers too. This is not an activity that is consigned to white men and women.'

Trans Remembrance Day

Intolerance sometimes leads to extreme violence. November 20th is the annual Transgender Remembrance Day which pays tribute to people across the world who have been murdered simply because they are trans. The number of transgender murders is staggeringly high in South American countries, with trans people sometimes battered to death. The highest numbers of recorded murders are in Brazil, Mexico and Colombia. Outside Central and South America the most murders of trans people recorded are in the USA, Turkey and the Philippines. However, even Europe is not free of transphobic violence: numbers recorded by Press for Change (the UK's transgender activist group, www.pfc.org.uk) for a immigration tribunal found that between 1999 and 2015, nine trans people had been homicide victims in the UK, but more than 50 had been murdered in Italy in the same period. Most of the Italian victims were immigrants and working as sex workers. This highlights the need for gender recognition and equality legislation. In Italy, the law does not enable trans people to even change their name, never mind their legal gender, until they have undergone genital reconstructive surgery. There is only one Gender Identity Clinic in Italy providing free access to gender reassignment treatments, compared with ten NHS Clinics in the UK.

Tara, trans woman. 'These hate crimes in South America are appalling, with innocent people battered to death every year for being trans. It is evil and cruel, with its roots, I believe, firmly sown in ignorance. Many of these crimes are committed in areas of poverty with the perpetrators coming from the same lower social economic backgrounds as the victims. Every year on Trans Remembrance Day, I pray for the victims, and for these killings to end. I believe those murdered are shining their light down on us and giving us the courage and willpower to continue living as open trans people.

What happens in South America – and indeed America itself – is far worse than what we experience in Europe. Despite there being discrimination and prejudice in abundance at times, things are generally good. I do believe the world is becoming a much better place for trans people as a whole.

I know I am one of the lucky ones because I have never been attacked or threatened with violence. Maybe this is because I transitioned when I was 17 and pass well as a woman. I go about my business without fear and, apart from the occasional stare or comment here and there, I largely live a normal life. I know a lot of other trans women though who are older, and maybe do not pass as convincingly as I do, who have endured suffering and harassment.

But I can tell you they are such kind souls who have not become bitter as a result of their experiences. They have a good attitude about themselves and about life. They give off a good energy and are lovely people to know and to be around.

This is all part of the trans beauty which people, including trans people themselves, need to embrace more. Whether you are a trans man or a trans woman – does it matter whether you pass as either? Surely, what matters most is what is in your heart and how you interact with other people.'

Community violence and intimidation

The level of violence against trans people is still a problem in Europe and the UK, despite European Equality directives and case law which require countries in Europe to provide humane gender recognition legislation. Harassment is sometimes close to home. A lot of trans people experience discrimination and fear violence in their local neighbourhood, be it on ordinary streets or council estates. In these situations, life remains difficult for people who face ridicule, ostracism, physical threats, intimidation or silent harassment and sometimes violence for being trans.

Elodie, trans woman. 'I still sometimes get hostility in my local area. I've had my front door kicked in several times by people who previously lived next door to me. Maybe they saw me as a threat. Thankfully, my current neighbours are more tolerant. Rude remarks in my local area are frequent but you get used to them. Wolf whistles I can tolerate, because they are more humorous than malicious. I used to keep indoors a lot to avoid ridicule but I discovered there is far less fear if I venture out dressed as a female every few days rather than leaving it for several weeks.'

Megan, trans woman. 'Be as confident as you can. Confidence breeds confidence. Don't let idiots knock you back. I remember being in a shopping mall once and heard the words "Freak, Freak!", knowing only too well that they were being directed at me. I made sure I went out the next day. I felt nervous and highly-strung, but it was something I had to prove to myself, that I could beat the bullies. These days I no longer walk around with my head bowed. I look straight at people. I meet their eyes and as a result very little abuse is directed at me.'

Jean, trans woman. 'Trans women bring up emotional issues in heterosexual men. I mean men who like to portray themselves as a superman, Jack the lad or the gym types who love their muscles. They see a pretty woman in the street but when she looks around they discover that it is a trans and not a cisgender woman. They start questioning themselves and wonder if they really fancied a man who happened to be wearing a dress. After a quick internalising of the situation, their thoughts turn to anger and revulsion against themselves, which often results in violence towards the person that they had fancied moments beforehand.'

Certain strands of society and the media hold a preoccupation with transition and surgery, and fail to focus on other aspects of the person's life. This places great emotional strain on people who are expected to conform to the expectations of others. Until very recently, the unemployment rate amongst the trans community, particularly trans women, was quite high. This was unjust and minimised the life experiences and skills of some well-educated people who come from many different occupations with many skills to offer, if given the chance.

Although trans issues have come a long way from where they were in the past few decades, the main issues that affect trans people remain the same: direct discrimination, abuse, violence, as well as hostility and insensitivity from healthcare providers. For example, there are those who ask trans people what their previous name was before they transitioned (under the guise of completing paperwork). Even young people are sometimes cruel. This brings up the issue of trans education in schools: why are young children not taught about these nuances of gender and sexuality?

Felicity, trans woman. 'I live opposite a school. Some of the students throw things at me and my friends when they see us walking past. I went into the school once to report it. "We won't stand for that type of behaviour", announced the Principal, but I never heard back from him and the conduct did not improve, leaving me to believe that nothing was done about it. I have spoken at conferences about transgender issues, even at a police training school, but I would be loath to go into a school to give a talk because I genuinely fear being laughed at and mocked. Faith schools, I imagine, wouldn't even entertain the idea of a trans person entering their doors. But I know it is education and awareness that is needed.

I was walking down a street recently with my partner and two other trans friends when we encountered a man on the opposite side with his two children, both under the age of six. The man alerted the children of our presence and started pointing and laughing at us. The children stared and laughed at what their father was saying. You wonder what chance these kids have got. This is how transphobia is bred.'

Benson, trans man. 'I remember being out walking with a trans female friend, who was in the early stages of transition, one evening in summertime. Suddenly, we heard a child shout "Fucking tranny!" before he suddenly rode his bike into us, injuring my friend in the leg. Here was a young boy who was out intentionally to cause harm. We later wondered if he was the product of what he heard at home; somewhere that made him learn to hate trans people, gay people or anybody else who was different. We didn't bother reporting it to the police because they do not really recognise transphobia as a crime. The most it would get recorded as would be a hate crime.'

Enquiring into somebody's transition status or whether they have legal gender recognition – for example, asking if they are pre- or post-op – is not only in bad taste but also shows an ignorance in assuming that every trans person seeks to have reassignment surgery. Asking a trans person if they are trapped in the wrong body and how they feel about this is also considered intrusive. Likewise, with sexuality, it is best not to make generalisations. Trans men are not always looking for a female partner and neither are trans women always looking for a male partner. There is a whole range of possibilities, as you will have read in the chapter on sexuality, and it is best not to ask personal questions without getting to know the person first, and only then upon invitation.

Seiran, non-binary. 'The case of misgendering comes up all the time. I was in the early days of my hormone treatment and my voice hadn't yet broken. I was at a low ebb in my life when I applied for disability allowance. I hadn't worked for months due to depression and needed some financial support. The woman on the other end of the line asked, "Are you married or divorced?" "Neither", I replied, being placed in a situation where I had to explain that I was a trans man and the reason for the different name/ gender on my birth certification was that I changed my name legally by deed poll. The woman burst out laughing and continued to giggle intermittently before putting down the receiver.'

Terry, non-binary. 'Discrimination is commonplace and sometimes resembles homophobia. One day I was in a restaurant holding hands with my girlfriend, when we overheard another woman at a nearby table go out of her way to disturb our peace by loudly saying, for us to hear her, "They shouldn't be allowed to do that!"'

Ria, trans woman. 'The worst piece of discrimination that I experienced came from a childhood friend who I have known all my life. We were really close and she was one of the first people I came out to. I hadn't expected her reaction. The hatred just flowed out of her. The words "faggot" and "paedophile" lingered in my mind for days, weeks and months afterwards. They wouldn't leave me. It was torture. We were two people who had always got on well together, but she was prepared to cast me aside like I was meaningless to her. It still hurts.'

Dara, trans woman. 'I remember being on a train. There were three teenage boys in a row of seats behind me giggling. They let off a fire extinguisher and sprayed the hose in my direction before chanting, "Batty man!" The guard was kind. He ordered the boys to move to another carriage and got me some tissues to dry myself.'

Melissa, trans woman. 'Every person has different experiences and life conditions and although transition with surgical intervention is the ultimate goal for some trans people, it is not possible for everyone. Indeed, there are different medical, psychological and social barriers for every person to transition. This sometimes results in a split within the trans community when preferences and experiences differ to others.'

Stan, trans man. 'I was once on a weekend training programme to become a mentor for young LGBT people when I overheard some other men on the course making a joke about trans women. This meant I had to out myself before telling them that what they were saying was totally unacceptable. I questioned their suitability for potentially mentoring young trans people. They failed to acknowledge their ignorance or to apologise.'

Another prejudice that comes to the forefront is directed towards non-binary people, often from within the trans community itself. Some trans women and trans men claim that opinions of non-binaries don't count because they have not lived through the harsh experiences they've had to endure (like taking hormone therapies or having surgery to be considered a proper trans person). This is not fair, and incorrect if you consider that some non-binary people do choose to have hormone therapy and undergo surgeries.

Reid, non-binary. 'It is not uncommon to be told, I've fought tooth and nail to get where I am now. I appreciate the experiences of trans women in particular and the difficult time they must have had, but I too have had a tough time. I am taking a low dosage of testosterone to look more androgynous and to develop more body hair. I hate having to bind my breasts and although I don't want to completely remove my breasts, I am planning reduction surgery. In my experience, most non-binary people seek some type of medical intervention.

I have encountered other trans people who believe younger trans people are being let off far too lightly. They believe that medical and societal advancements rob people of the life experience of having to encounter discrimination which, they feel, helps shape a trans person to fight more passionately for equality. Then there are those who feel nobody has the right to call themselves trans unless that person has had full reassignment surgery.'

Another significant aspect of discrimination comes from television because there are still so very few trans people portrayed in the entertainment industry. So each portrayal is important, but until recently a large number of these portrayals were caricatures. Understandably, trans people are annoyed about the way they are featured in soaps and sitcoms; but an immense amount of work has been undertaken to alter this in recent years particularly by a UK charity called Trans Media Watch, which is a watchdog that helps people in the media to understand trans issues and produce clear, accurate, respectful material. There are currently a lot of good drama and documentary programmes in production which will see some very positive progress being made.

Lynne, trans woman. 'Any time a trans woman or cross-dresser is featured in a soap or sitcom, they are never portrayed as normal. There is always something wrong with them, as in the film *Psycho*. It seems that writers expect the viewers to want us to be weird and unpleasant. Other people think it is a sexual perversion and that sex always plays a part in it, which isn't the case.'

Simone, trans woman. 'Why doesn't the regulatory authority do something about advertisements on the television that portray trans people in demeaning and ill-advised ways? Would Ofcom allow black or disabled people to be mocked in this way? Tell me they wouldn't take action against this discrimination – yet for trans people, we are ignored, marginalised and forgotten.'

Farrell, trans man. 'We need more trans journalists. We need better media training for trans people. That way, we will be much better equipped at how best to portray ourselves in the media spotlight. Overall, the media needs to listen to trans people, take an interest in what their lives are about and, above all, be more responsible in their reportage. However, some trans people don't do themselves any favours. They sell their stories to newspapers and magazines for a few hundred pounds, but the financial reward can never undo the damage that is done. They are often taken advantage of and have their stories manipulated to suit the tabloid press. Usually this sets a negative tone that inadvertently sets trans people up to be attacked and mocked because they are viewed as fair game.'

Guy, trans man. 'A lot of trans people lose jobs, or find it difficult to get jobs. There is evidence that the earnings of a trans person are significantly lower than if they weren't trans. That is a further deterrent for them to seeking recompense. It actually pretty much prevents any trans person from pursuing any action against a newspaper in the courts.'

Equality Act 2010

In the UK, the Equality Act 2010 has made discrimination towards trans people unlawful in employment, and when accessing goods, services, housing and facilities – unless it can be demonstrated to be a reasonable means of pursuing a legitimate aim. There is an exception for single sex services, where protected characteristics exist for legitimate reasons. For example, a female rape counselling service can choose not to employ a trans person, although almost all of these services now have policies whereby they have chosen to be fair employers of trans people, and would employ a trans person who was appropriately qualified. The workplace, however, can still throw up all sorts of challenges for trans people, including those for colleagues who are likely never to have had direct contact with a trans person.

Vanessa, trans woman. 'Legislation in recent years has benefited the trans community more than ever before in history. But when it comes to getting a job, trans people are seen as a gamble, a weak link, because employers think that people will not take us seriously and will sneer at us as well as the employer for giving the job in the first place. Another major drawback is perceived mental instability because we are under the care of a psychiatrist.'

The law in the majority of Western countries states that a trans person should be able to use the toilet of their acquired gender without fear of harassment. If a non-transgender person objects to a trans person in the toilet, it is necessary for the employer to point out that toilets are available for use by everyone on the basis of their gender presentation, including trans people who intend to undergo, or are undergoing or have undergone a process or part of a process of gender reassignment.

Morgan, trans man. 'I am lucky that I have been in my job for a couple of years. I dread the prospect of having to find another job sometimes. There are always so many awkward questions around my documentation, my legal status and the way I present. Getting the point across to people that basically I am a man but that my passport identifies me as a woman is not always easy. Through ignorance, people often don't get some of the fundamental principles of what it is to be transgender. Bigoted people ensure that they make life as difficult as possible when you are in this situation.'

The Equality Act 2010 in the UK clearly sets out protective measures to safeguard transgender people and people closely associated to them from direct and indirect discrimination. It fully takes into consideration that transgender people need to take time off work to attend medical appointments and surgery and makes it unlawful for any employer to refuse requests for these purposes.

Imagine you arrive at work one morning and as you trawl through your emails you notice one from your boss informing the team that your colleague Paul, who is currently on holiday, has decided to change his gender and is to be addressed as Paula when she returns from holiday. You have been asked to respect Paula's privacy at the time and to acknowledge this momentous change in her life by granting her the support, respect and sensitivity that she deserves.

What do you think your initial reaction might be? Would you be surprised, astounded – or think that it is somebody's idea of a joke? You might stifle some giggles; you might nudge your friend next to you, drawing their attention to the email, but you don't know what your reaction might be unless you have been in a situation like this. Even though you have been asked to refer to Paula using female pronouns, you may still find that the name 'Paul' and male pronouns keep coming to your mind. You might question the quality of your friendship given you had not the slightest intimation that he wanted to become a woman. Lots of questions may flash through your mind as the morning progresses: how you will react when you see her? What you will say? You may wonder if you will feel comfortable sitting next to her. Paula may become the main focus of discussion during lunchtime and during coffee breaks. Of course, some colleagues will be kind and broadminded. Others less so, and may make cruel transphobic comments.

During the course of the day you may develop opinions and ideas in your head from what your colleagues have said that you might not otherwise have thought of before. When you get home, you might feel obliged to tell your spouse and children about Paula. After all, it's not every day this type of event happens at work. There might be humour and laughter. Your children may enquire what clothes Paula will be wearing when she presents to the office as a woman. They may even enquire what toilet she will use.

Thankfully, Paula has the law on her side. Direct discrimination in this instance would occur if a colleague did not want to sit next to Paula because she is trans. Indirect discrimination may occur if there was a rule or policy which put her at a particular disadvantage; for example, if Paula's company refused to change her email address to her new name, causing her the particular humiliation of being constantly outed by the email address which shows her previous name. Having laws in place is a great achievement but is it enough? Breaking down bias and prejudice is even better, so it's essential for as many non-trans people as possible to help bring about this change.

The Western world continues to be progressively liberal in LGBT issues. In the main, gay and lesbian people are readily accepted without hesitation across the world in a wide range of occupations because they are valued as being equal to everybody else. The days of widespread endemic homophobia are over. With regards to trans people, the journey is well under way to allow them to be as equally accepted and appreciated as everybody else. By the time another generation has passed, it's estimated that a large number of trans people will be a common feature in the workforce and will enjoy the same acceptance that gay and lesbian people currently do. That's not saying that there won't be difficult times for many trans people, nor will everyone be happy about it. But trans people aren't going to go away. In fact, the future will see the opposite occurring and this is simply something that transphobic people will need to get used to.

A few years ago Stonewall, the LGBT rights organisation, came up with a slogan, *Some people are gay. Get over it.* In the main, people in the Western world have got over it. More recently, they repeated their slogan for trans people. *Some people are trans. Get over it.* Indeed, the time has come to get over it. As I said at the beginning of this book, I consider myself to be an ally of trans people. So too can you be, whether you are part of the LGBT community or not. Can I encourage you all to welcome trans people into your lives with kindness and respect. Please don't let fear prevent you from making friends with a trans person because in doing so you could be missing out on meeting an extraordinary person.

Afterword

Jane Fae
Writer, feminist and campaigner for change

Trans Voices contains little that is absolutely new. How could it? The recent media focus on 'the trans experience' means we are subject as never before to a non-stop bombardment of trans stories, trans snippets and trans anecdotes.

Not all are well-informed. Still, we are a long way forward from even five years ago, when the press obsession was mostly with trans as strange, trans as abnormal, trans as a 'freak show'. Trans people are at last being heard, not as some amorphous mass, but as individuals. Caitlyn Jenner, Kellie Maloney, Janet Mock, Rebecca Root and a host of others. We have names and faces: and if the focus remains, for now, on trans women, that, too, will change.

So the long journey through the wilderness is over? Can those of us working for trans rights tip our virtual hats in the direction of a previous generation, including such stalwarts of the campaign for equality as Stephen Whittle and Christine Burns, and go home?

Well, not quite. Much has been done; yet much is still to do, and *Trans Voices* illustrates perfectly some of the gaps. To begin, it delivers precisely what it says on the label: these are trans voices – ordinary trans voices – talking about personal experience. This is important. For even the best of feature reporting tends toward shoe-boxing – the attempt to fit trans people into this or that cis/non-trans framework or issue.

Every story must have a beginning, middle and end; and while that may work well when it comes to selling papers, it is less helpful when it comes to communicating real experience. Less helpful, too, that the general media approach is to focus on soundbites taken from this or that famous person.

Which is why I enjoyed *Trans Voices*; for here, neatly arranged according to some of the primary divisions within the trans community – including the non-binary, of which we usually hear far less – are individual, unfamous trans people talking about their own lives. And although I began by suggesting that none of the parts were absolutely new, the effort invested in putting them together certainly is.

Because taken as a whole, the interviews, the personal statements, provide a richness and diversity to what it is to be trans. Here I echo what Stephen Whittle writes in his foreword to the book: *Being a trans activist...I am able to contribute to the discussions of trans people's issues, but I am not some sort of trans person representative.*

I thank my lucky stars that unlike Shirley, talking of her experience in the '60s, I was never threatened *with heavy psychotropic drugs, then electro shock therapy, and finally lobotomy.* Reading on, I found myself alternately nodding in agreement or, less often, bridling slightly at some commentary I did not agree with.

But agree or disagree, I recognised each and every point of view as ones that I have encountered in my various journeys around the trans community; as I have come to realise that (Stephen Whittle again): *I am just one of many types of trans people, I lead just one sort of trans person's life.*

Yes, yes and yes again! We are not all the same. We are not some homogenous mass in which one trans stands for every trans.

Important, too, were the hints here and there that the trans project, by which I mean no more than the struggle for equal rights before the law, remains unfinished. Medical and psychiatric attitudes have improved much over the last couple of decades, but they remain less than perfect; and the nuts and bolts of medical support are still random, haphazardly supported.

Meanwhile, in broader legislative terms, being trans means continuing to suffer under a form of State discrimination that has much in common with the discrimination by which the State once accorded different rights according to one's gender or racial status.

Trans people still do not have the same rights as non-trans people. Our very existence is defined and judged by 'experts' who are not trans; our protests, when we do protest, are dismissed as extreme or ungrateful.

Which is why, to return to the beginning, we need to hear trans voices more than ever: to understand the diversity of trans people; to understand the similarities and, too, the differences between us; above all, to go beyond the idea that anyone who is not trans can ever really get what it is to be trans.

Glossary

Androphilic – sexual attraction to men or masculinity.

Assigned at birth – a phrase used by trans men, trans women and non-binary people to describe the inadvertent mistake that was made about their gender identity when they were born.

Binding – flattening the chest to create the external appearance of a male torso.

Cisgender – a synonym for non-trans people. It comes from the Latin cis meaning on the same side and is used to describe someone who is comfortable in the gender they were assigned at birth.

Cross-dresser – one who adopts the clothes, appearance and behaviour normally associated with the opposite gender. The person usually identifies with the gender assigned at birth. The majority of cross-dressers describe their sexual orientation as heterosexual (see also transvestite).

Drag kings – are women, usually lesbian, who dress in masculine clothes and often act with exaggerated masculinity and in male gender roles for comic, dramatic or satirical effect.

Drag queens – are men, usually gay, who dress in female clothes and often act with exaggerated femininity and in female gender roles for comic, dramatic or satirical effect.

DSM – *The Diagnostic and Statistical Manual of Mental Disorders*, published by the American Psychiatric Association; offers a common language and standard criteria for the classification of mental disorders.

Female to male (FTM) – an individual assigned female at birth but whose gender identity is male.

Facial feminisation surgery (FFS) – is a set of reconstructive surgical procedures that alter typically male facial features to bring them closer in shape and size to typical female facial features.

Gender dysphoria – psychiatric term most commonly used in America and most parts of Europe, UK and Ireland to describe a trans person who feels the gender assigned to them at birth is incongruent with their brain, which tells them they are the opposite gender – or both genders – or does not correlate as either gender.

Gender expression – how a person displays/portrays their gender to others through dress and/or societal gender roles.

Gender identity disorder – a previous classification given to trans people who expressed a desire to transition to the opposite gender of their birth. Now mainly referred to as gender dysphoria in the Western world and the majority of Europe.

Gender identity – is a person's internal feeling of being male, female or some other gender or combination of genders. Gender identity is completely separate from an individual's sexual orientation.

Gender reassignment surgery (GRS) – also known as genital reconstruction surgery or gender confirmation surgery. It is the procedure (or procedures) by which a trans person's physical appearance and function of their existing sexual characteristics are altered to accord with their identified gender, including genital surgery. Not all trans people undergo surgery for a variety of social, medical and personal reasons. The colloquial term 'sex change' is offensive to trans people.

GIC – Gender Identity Clinic. Specialist NHS services in the UK, run by consultant psychiatrists, providing assessment for trans people who are seeking hormone treatment and/or surgical gender reassignment procedures.

Gynephilic – sexual attraction to women or femininity.

Intersex – There are over 40 known intersex variations, but a simplistic explanation is that intersex people have chromosomal incongruities and are born with visibly ambiguous genitalia that do not entirely fit that of what is considered male or female.

Male to female (MTF) – an individual assigned male at birth but whose gender identity is female.

Misgendering – this term refers to a trans person and relates to somebody using a word, especially a pronoun or form of address (whether deliberate or accidental) that does not correctly reflect the gender with which they identify.

Non-binary – not part of the man/woman gender binary model. The binary model is limiting because it has room for only two categories, and those categories must be opposites as man or woman.

Purge – a term that cross-dressers use to describe their inner disdain at themselves, which results in them disposing of all their clothes in a bid to free themselves from their internalised guilt and shame.

Packing – a bought or homemade accoutrement to create the external appearance of male genitalia.

Pansexual – somebody who is sexually attracted to all types of gender including cisgender men and women, trans men and trans women and non-binary people.

Real life experience (RLE) – an outdated process that used to be imposed on trans people seeking hormone medication. It has been replaced by a fixed period of 12 months living in the new gender role before trans people can be eligible for genital surgery.

Stealth – passing as non-trans without revealing your trans status.

Trans – an umbrella term for people whose gender identity and/or gender expression diverges in some way from the sex they were assigned at birth, including those who identify as transsexual people, those who identify as non-binary gender people, and cross-dressing people.

Trans man (FTM) – the usual term to describe female to male trans people but does not apply to all trans people who see themselves as being towards the masculine end of the gender spectrum. Another definition is a person who was assigned female at birth but has a male gender identity and therefore proposes to transition, is transitioning or has transitioned to live as a man, often with the assistance of hormone treatment and perhaps various surgical procedures.

Trans woman (MTF) – the usual term to describe male to female trans people but does not apply to all trans people who see themselves as being towards the feminine end of the gender spectrum. Another definition is a person who was assigned male at birth but has a female gender identity and therefore proposes to transition, is transitioning or has transitioned to live as a woman, often with the assistance of hormone treatment and perhaps various surgical procedures.

Transgender – often used as an alternative word to transsexual, it is also used by some as longhand word for trans and an umbrella term that is used to describe someone who does not conform to society's view of being male or female. It can be used to mean a variety of gender identities and expressions, as in non-binary people (see transsexual).

Transition – the process of becoming the gendered person you know yourself to be.

Transphobia – a fear, dislike or intolerance directed towards trans people, or a fear or dislike directed towards their perceived lifestyle, culture or characteristics, whether or not any specific trans person has that lifestyle or characteristic.

Transsexual – is an acute form of gender dysphoria where a person's perception of their gender is opposite to their biological sex. It is a medical term used to describe people whose sex and gender do not match up. This means someone whose biological sex is male but whose gender identity is a woman, or someone whose biological sex is female but whose gender identity is a man. Transsexual people may feel as if they were born in the wrong body (see transgender).

Transvestite – a term that has been around since the 1930s, used to describe people who dress in clothes associated with the opposite gender. They usually identify with the gender they were assigned at birth and are mainly heterosexual (see also cross-dresser).

WPATH – Formerly known as the Harry Benjamin International Gender Dysphoria Association (HBIGDA), WPATH is a non-profit, interdisciplinary professional and educational organisation devoted to transgender health. It consists of professional and student members who engage in clinical and academic research to develop evidence-based medicine and strive to promote a high quality of care for transsexual, transgender and gender-nonconforming individuals internationally. It is funded primarily through the support of its membership and through donations and grants sponsored by non-commercial sources.

References

American Psychiatric Association. (2013) *Diagnostic and Statistical Manual of Mental Disorders (DSM-5)*. Washington, DC: American Psychiatric Association.

Amnesty International. (2014) *The State Decides Who I Am*. London: Amnesty International.

Baron-Cohen, S. and Jones, M. R. (2011) 'Female-to-male transsexual people and autistic traits.' *Journal of Autism and Developmental Disorders*, (Issue 42) 30 March 2011, 301–6. Dillon, M. (1946) *Self: A Study in Ethics and Endocrinology*. Amsterdam: Elsevier Science.

Green, J. (2004) *Becoming a Visible Man*. Nashville, TN: Vanderbilt University Press.

Hall, R. (2008) *The Well of Loneliness*. London: Virago; reprint edition (originally published 1928).

Lips, H. M. (2014) *Gender: The Basics*. London: Routledge.

McNeil, J. Bailey, L. Ellis, S. Morton, J. and Regan, M. (2012) *Trans Mental Health Study*. Sheffield: Sheffield Hallam University.

McNeil, J. Bailey, L. Ellis, S. and Regan, M. (2013) *Speaking from the Margins: Trans Mental Health and Wellbeing in Ireland*. Ireland: Transgender Equality Network Ireland (TENI).

Pace Charity. (2014) *The RaRE Research Report: LGB&T Mental Health - Risk and Resilience Explored*. London: PACE Charity UK.

World Health Organization. (2012) *The International Statistical Classification of Diseases and Health Related Problems (ICD-10)*. Geneva: World Health Organization.

Zhou, J-N. Hofman, M. A. Gooren, L. J. and Swaab, L. J. (1995) *A Sex Difference in the Human Brain and its Relation to Transsexuality*. Amsterdam: Netherlands Institute for Brain Research.

Further Reading

Belge, K. and Bieschke, M. (2011) *Queer: The Ultimate LGBT Guide for Teens.* San Francisco, CA: Zest Books.

Boyd, H. (2007) *She's Not the Man I Married: My Life with a Transgender Husband.* Berkeley, CA: Seal Press.

Brown, L. M. and Rounsley, C. A. (1996) *Understanding Transsexualism.* San Francisco, CA: Jossey-Bass.

Herman, J. (2009) *Transgender Explained.* Bloomington, IN: Author House.

McBride, R-S. (2013) *Grasping the Nettle: the Experiences of Gender Variant Children and Transgender Youth Living in Northern Ireland.* Belfast: Institute of Conflict Research.

Terrence Higgins Trust. (2012) *Trans Men (Sexual Health, HIV and Wellbeing – A Guide for Trans Men).* London: Terrence Higgins Trust.

Terrence Higgins Trust. (2012) *Trans Women (Sexual Health, HIV and Wellbeing – A Guide for Trans Women).* London: Terrence Higgins Trust.

Useful Contacts

Here is a list of some key organisations in the UK and Ireland that lend support and guidance to trans people and their families. They are mainly national organisations, or those better known to trans people, but the list is by no means an exhaustive one. These contacts are not intended to deter any person seeking further information or support from their nearest LGBT organisation. Please note some of the contacts listed here may only be contacted via their website and/or by telephone and not all of them have a postal address.

Britain

Gendered Intelligence is a community interest company who works predominantly with the trans community and those who impact on trans lives. They particularly specialise in supporting young trans people aged 8–25. They also deliver trans youth programmes, support for parents and carers, professional development and trans awareness training for all sectors and educational workshops for schools, colleges, universities and other educational settings.

> **Gendered Intelligence**
> 200a Pentonville Road
> London
> N1 9JP
> Telephone: 0207 832 5848
> Website: www.genderedintelligence.co.uk

Gender Identity Research and Education Society (GIRES) is a national organisation which was set up to improve the lives of trans and gender non-conforming people, including those who are non-binary and non-gender.

> **The Gender Identity Research and Education Society (GIRES)**
> Melverley
> The Warren
> Ashtead
> Surrey
> KT21 2SP
> Telephone: 01372 801554
> Website: www.gires.org.uk

The Beaumont Society is a UK self-help body run by and for the transgender community. They welcome all transgender people and their partners, regardless of gender, sexual orientation, race, creed or colour and all varieties from the nervous newcomers to those who are experienced and confident in their preferred gender.

> **The Beaumont Society**
> 27 Old Gloucester Street
> London
> WC1N 3XX
> Telephone: 01582 412220
> Email: enquiries@beaumontsociety.org.uk
> Website: www.beaumontsociety.org.uk

UK Trans Info is a national charity focused on improving the lives of trans and non-binary people in the UK.

> **UK Trans Info**
> PO Box 871
> 109 Vernon House
> Friar Lane
> Nottingham
> NG1 6DQ
> Email: info@uktrans.info
> Website: www.uktrans.info

Trans Media Watch is a charity dedicated to improving media coverage of trans and intersex issues. They aim to assist people in the media to understand these issues and produce clear, accurate, respectful material. It also helps trans and intersex people who are interacting with the media to get results they are comfortable with.

> **Trans Media Watch**
> London
> WC1N 3XX
> Website: www.transmediawatch.org

Press for Change is a key lobbying and legal support organisation for trans people in the UK. They provide legal advice, training, and research to trans people, their representatives, and public and private bodies.

Press For Change
BM Network
London
WC1N 3XX
Telephone: 0844 8708165
Email: office@pfc.org.uk
Website: www.pfc.org.uk

The National Trans Youth Network is a network of trans youth groups across the UK. They represent young trans people up to the age of 25 across all areas of the UK, with groups from England, Scotland, Wales and Northern Ireland.

The National Trans Youth Network
Website: www.ntyn.org.uk

Mermaids are a UK charity set up by a group of parents whose children experienced gender identity issues. It has evolved and grown to meet demand and offer appropriate resources to young people, up to the age of 19, their families and carers, and professionals working with gender variant young people.

Mermaids
BM Mermaids
London
WC1N 3XX
Telephone: 0844 3340550
Website: www.mermaidsuk.org.uk

Wales

LGBT Cymru Helpline offers a free and professional caring service for transgender people in Wales aiming to offer support and information to the trans men, trans women, non-binary – partners, parents and families and friends. They offer a free telephone helpline and a low cost counselling service.

LGBT Cymru Helpline
c/o 92 Corporation Avenue
Llanelli
Wales
SA15 3SR
Telephone: 0800 840 2069
Website: www.lgbtcymruhelpline.org.uk

Scotland

Scottish Transgender Alliance assists transgender people, service providers, employers and equality organisations to engage together to improve gender identity and gender reassignment equality, rights and inclusion in Scotland. They strive for everyone in Scotland to be safe and valued whatever their gender identity and gender reassignment status and to have full freedom in their gender expression.

> **Scottish Transgender Alliance**
> Equality Network
> 30 Bernard Street
> Edinburgh
> EH6 6PR
> Telephone: 0131 467 6039
> Email: sta@equality-network.org
> Website: www.scottishtrans.org

Transgender Support Programmes within LGBT Health provide social groups, confidence building workshops and one-to-one support for transgender people.

> **Transgender Support Programmes**
> LGBT Health and Wellbeing
> 9 Howe Street
> Edinburgh
> EH3 6TE
> Telephone: 0131 523 1100
> Email: admin@lgbthealth.org.uk
> Website: www.lgbthealth.org.uk

Northern Ireland

Transgender Northern Ireland is a website that provides general information, advice and confidential support in many areas of life and around various issues that people might experience. Their qualified staff and trained volunteers are able to help any caller with gender identity issues.

> Website: www.transgenderni.com

GenderJam is a community group for the young transgender community in Northern Ireland, based mostly in the Belfast area. They bring young transgender, non-binary, questioning and intersex people together and create resources to help the community in Northern Ireland. They also provide individual support for young people experiencing difficulty with housing, education, healthcare and other issues that affect the trans community in the region.

GenderJam NI
Belfast LGBT Centre
9-13 Waring Street
Belfast
BT1 2DX
Telephone: 028 90 996 819
Website: www.genderjam.org.uk

Republic of Ireland

Transgender Equality Network Ireland (TENI) is the leading trans organisation in Ireland who seeks to improve conditions and advance the rights and equality of trans people and their families throughout the Republic of Ireland.

Transgender Equality Network Ireland (TENI)
Unit 2
4 Ellis Quay
Dublin 7
Ireland
Telephone: 00353+ (01) 873 3575
Email: info@teni.ie
Website: www.teni.ie

Index